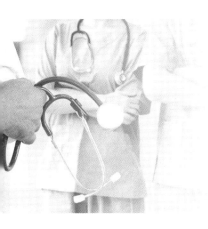

医院管理学
常用词录

张鹭鹭 丁陶 张寓景 主编

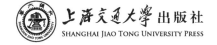

上海交通大学出版社
SHANGHAI JIAO TONG UNIVERSITY PRESS

内容提要

本书广泛收集了4000余条医院管理及相关学科领域实用词汇和近年来出现的一些新词汇。内容既涉及传统医院管理范畴,如医疗质量管理、医疗安全管理、医院感染管理、医院财务管理及医院信息管理等;又包含了医院管理领域的最新进展,如医院战略管理、医院资本运营管理、医院质量认证、医院知识管理、公立医院产权制度改革、医疗资源配置、药品流通改革与医院管理、社区卫生服务与医院管理、医院管理新方法等;同时还收集了相关学科,如社会医学、卫生统计学、卫生经济学、流行病学及卫生法学的部分词汇。

本书可供各级卫生机关领导干部及其他卫生工作人员、医院管理者、从事卫生事业管理教学与理论研究者、医院管理研究工作者、翻译人员和医药卫生事业相关专业工作者学习参考。

图书在版编目(CIP)数据

医院管理学常用词录 / 张鹭鹭,丁陶,张寓景主编.
—上海:上海交通大学出版社,2021.11
ISBN 978 - 7 - 313 - 25490 - 0

Ⅰ.①医… Ⅱ.①张… ②丁… ③张… Ⅲ.①医院-管理学-词汇-汇编 Ⅳ.①R197.32 - 61

中国版本图书馆 CIP 数据核字(2021) 第 191865 号

医院管理学常用词录
YIYUAN GUANLIXUE CHANGYONG CILU

主　　编:张鹭鹭　丁　陶　张寓景
出版发行:上海交通大学出版社　　　　地　　址:上海市番禺路 951 号
邮政编码:200030　　　　　　　　　　电　　话:021 - 64071208
印　　刷:常熟市文化印刷有限公司　　经　　销:全国新华书店
开　　本:710mm×1000mm　1/16　　印　　张:16
字　　数:234 千字
版　　次:2021 年 11 月第 1 版　　　　印　　次:2021 年 11 月第 1 次印刷
书　　号:ISBN 978 - 7 - 313 - 25490 - 0
定　　价:98.00 元

《医院管理学常用词录》
编译人员名单

主　审　陈　洁

主　编　张鹭鹭　丁　陶　张寓景

编　委　（以姓氏笔画为序）

丁　陶　王　君　王露尧　卢　杨

叶　锋　刘　旭　刘　源　吴　强

张　义　张　宇　张寓景　张鹭鹭

陆　琳　欧崇阳　郝　璐　胡友花

胡超群　栗美娜　唐碧菡　康　鹏

潘禹安　薛　晨　戴志鑫　戴鲁男

使 用 说 明

一、本词录由英汉、汉英两部分组成。

二、排列方法

    1.英汉部分各词条均按英文字母顺序排列。

    2.汉英部分各词条均按汉语拼音字母顺序排列,同音异调的汉字按声调
        顺序排列,同音同调的汉字排列顺序与《新华字典》排列顺序相同。

三、符号用法

    1.圆括号:表示对该词条的缩写。

        例如:coronary care unit（UUC）　冠心病监护病房

    2.分号：表示英文(中文)词语不同的中译(英译)。

        例如：报酬 returns；reward

            drug abuse　滥用药物；吸毒

前　　言

随着国家和军队医疗卫生体制改革的不断推进,引领医院管理理论研究与实践探索逐步走向深入,医院管理及相关专业领域的文献与日俱增,新术语、新词汇不断涌现。了解和掌握这些新词汇对医院管理工作者做好本职工作和探索、研究卫生管理事业无疑是有益的。特别是随着科研成果及学术论文的交流日益国际化,期刊也大多要求撰写英文摘要和关键词。为适用广大医院管理及相关专业人员熟悉掌握和规范运用医院管理相关专业的中、英文词汇,准确地进行学术交流,我们编写了这本《医院管理学常用词录》工具书。

本书广泛收集了4 000余条医院管理及相关学科领域实用词汇和近年来出现的一些新词汇。内容既涉及传统医院管理范畴,如医疗质量管理、医疗安全管理、医院感染管理、医院财务管理及医院信息管理等;又包含了医院管理领域的最新进展,如医院战略管理、医院资本运营管理、医院质量认证、医院知识管理、公立医院产权制度改革、医疗资源配置、药品流通改革与医院管理、社区卫生服务与医院管理、医院管理新方法等;同时还收集了相关学科,如社会医学、卫生统计学、卫生经济学、流行病学及卫生法学的部分词汇。

本书可供各级卫生机关领导干部及其他卫生工作人员、医院管理者、从事卫生事业管理教学与理论研究者、医院管理研究工作者、翻译人员和医药卫生事业相关专业工作者学习参考。

本书在编写过程中得到了海军军医大学首长和机关的大力支持,军队卫生事业管理研究所的工作人员及研究生做了大量细致的工作。书稿完成后承蒙复旦大学医学院公共卫生学院陈洁教授审校,在此我们深表谢意。

尽管笔者收集词汇时尽可能采用多个蓝本相互核对,清样反复校对,但由于我们编写水平有限,本书难免存在不足之处,敬请读者批评指正。

主编

2021 年 6 月

目　　录

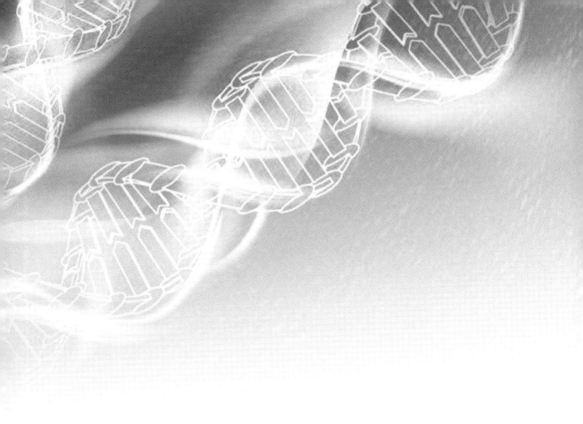

上 篇

英文—中文对照词汇

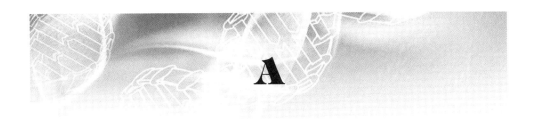

A

a deficit budgets　赤字预算

a minimum standard of living for city residents　城镇居民最低生活保障

a principle of maintaining a balance between revenues and expenditures　财政收支平衡原则

a proactive employment policy　积极的就业政策

a proactive fiscal policy　积极财政政策

a zero-base budgeting system　零基预算制度

ABC management method　ABC管理法

ability analysis　能力分析

ability to service debt　财政偿还能力

abnormal profit　不正常利润

abolish　废止

abridged life table　简略寿命表

absolute advantage　绝对优势

absorbed dose　吸收剂量

abstention　弃权

academicalism　唯学历论

acceptability　可接受性

acceptance inspection　验收检验

accessibility　可及性

account　核算

account book　会计账簿

account decision　财务决策

account settled　决算

accounting standard　会计准则

accounting statement　会计报表

accounts payable　应付账款

accreditation　认可

accreditation of medical staff　医务人员认证

accreditation of testing laboratories　认可实验室

accreditation period　评审周期

accreditation procedure　评审程序

accredited laboratory test report　实验室认可报告

accrediting body　认可机构

accrediting criteria　认可标准

accumulated depreciation　累积折旧

accumulated profit or loss　累积
盈亏

achievement　成果

achievement application　成果应用

achievement evaluation　业绩考评

achievement-oriented leader　成就
取向型领导

achievements in basic theory　基础
理论成果

acquisition　购买

action emending　行为修正

active follow-up　主动随访

active immunity　人工自动免疫

active management　主动管理

activeness　主动性

actual frequency　实际频数

actuarial method　保险精算法

actuarial science　保险精算学

actuary　精算师、保险统计员

adapt to demand　适应需求

adaptive randomization　适应性分组

additional premium　附加保险费

adjusted means　修正均数

administration cost　管理费

administration frequency　用药频度

administrative achievements　政绩

administrative command　行政指令

administrative department　机关职
能部门

administrative duty　行政职务

administrative enforcement　行政强
制执行

administrative intervention　行政
干预

administrative law　行政法

administrative management（ADM）
行政管理

administrative method　行政手段

administrative penalty in respect of
health　卫生行政处罚

administrative punishment　行政
处分

administrative staff　行政人员

admitting office　住院处

advantage　优势

adverse drug reaction　药物不良
反应

adverse drug reactions monitoring
药品不良反应监测

adverse effect　副作用

adverse event　不良事件

adverse reaction　不良反应

adverse selection　逆选择

advice for the patient; doctor's orders 医嘱

aeger 医师诊断证明书

aetiology 病因学

affiliation 归属

affiliation needs 归属的需要

affordability 可承受性

age group 年龄组

age structure 年龄结构

agency 代理处；机构

agency revenue 业务收入

agency stage 行政机关的裁决

agendum; operating instruction; operating manual 操作规程

age-sex composition 年龄性别组成

age-specific death rate 年龄别死亡率

aggregate demand 总需求

aggregate supply 总供给

aging of population 人口老龄化

agreement validity 一致性效度

agricultural economics 农业经济

aid station 救护所

aid station deployment 救护所部署

aid station on sea beach 滩头救护所

air force hospital 空军医院

alcohol abuse 酒精(乙醇)滥用

alcoholism 酒精依赖

allocation 分布；分配

allocation efficiency 配置效率

allocation index 配置指标

allocation procedure 配置程序

allocative efficiency 配置效率

alternative hypothesis 备选假设

alternative project 备选方案

altruistic value 利他价值

ambidirectional study 双向研究

ambispective cohort study 双向性队列研究

ambulance 救护车

ambulatory nursing 门诊护理

ambulatory nursing management 门诊护理管理

amendment 修订

American Association of Medical Colleges 美国医学院协会

American Joint Commission International Accreditation Standards for Hospitals 美国医疗机构评审联合委员会国际部医院评审标准

American National Standard Institute 美国国家标准机构

American Society for Quality 美国质量学会

American Society for Quality Control 美国质量控制学会

amortization 分期偿还

amount insured 保险金

analgesia mortality 手术麻醉死亡率

analog code 模拟编码

analog computation 模拟计算

analog control 模拟控制

analog data 模拟数据

analog display 模拟显示

analog network 模拟网络

analog psychology 模拟心理学

analog quantity 模拟量

analog signal 模拟信号

analog simulation 相似模拟

analog system 模拟系统

analogize 类似推理

analogue computer 模拟计算机

analogue digital conversion 模拟数字转换

analogue method 模拟法

analogue model 模拟模型

analogue technique 模拟技术

analogue transmission 模拟传输

analogy method of forecast 类推预测法

analogy test 模拟测验

analysis of casualties 减员分析

analysis of covariance 协方差分析

analysis of extremes 极限分析

analysis of multiple covariance 多元协方差分析

analysis of variance(ANOVA) 方差分析

analytical hierarchy process 层次分析法

anatomy 解剖学

anesthetist 麻醉师

animal experiment 动物实验

animal toxin 动物毒素

animal trial 动物试验

annual assessment 年度考核

annual average expense for equipment 设备年平均费用

annual growth rate 年增长率

annual increment of the population 每年人口增加数

annual net equivalent 年净当量

annual plan 年度计划

annual premium 年保险费

annual report of medical statistics

卫生统计年报

anthropogenic   人为污染

anti-infection drugs   抗感染药物

antishock group   抗休组

appeal   上诉

appease   抚慰

appellant   上诉人

applicability   适用性

applicant   申请人，参保人

applicant unit   参保单位

application   申请

application for clinical trial   临床研究申请

application of normative document   标准文件的应用

appointed evacuation   指定性后送

appraisal   鉴定

appraisal tool；evaluation tool   评价工具

appropriateness   适宜性

appropriateness evaluation   适宜性评价

appropriate rapid economic growth   经济适度快速增长

appropriation   无偿调拨

approval   批准

approval stage   批准阶段

arbitrage   无风险套利

arbitration   仲裁

architecture standard for hospital   医院建筑标准

area sampling   地区抽样

army hospital   部队医院

arrangement of health service   卫勤部署

art of leadership   领导艺术

Arthritis Impact Measurement Scale（AIMC）   关节炎影响量表

artificial intelligence（AI）   人工智能

artificial system   人工系统

asepsis section   无菌区

aseptic technique   无菌技术

Asian Standard Advisory Committee   亚洲标准咨询委员会

ask for instructions   请示

assessment   评估

assessment of conformity   评定合格

assessment of prefecture   任期考核

asset management   资产管理

assets   资产

assets leased to others   出租资产

assistant decision-making   辅助决策

assistant diagnosis and treat

department 辅助诊疗部门

assistant doctor 医士

assistant engineer 助理工程师

assistant equipment 辅助设备

assistant personnel 助理员

assistant pharmacist 药士；助理
药师

associate chief pharmacist 副主任
药师

associate professor 副教授

association 关联

assume responsibility for own profit
and loss 自负盈亏

assumption 假定

assurance of conformity 合格保证

asymmetric information 非对称性
信息

asymmetric information 信息不
对称

atmosphere 氛围

attack 发作

attenuation 弱化

attitude 态度

attributable proportion of interaction
交互作用归因比

attributable risk 归因危险度

attributable risk percent 归因危险

度百分比

audit 审核；审计

audit client 审核委托人

audit conclusion 审核结论

audit quality of care 医疗质量评鉴

auditing target 评估对象

auditing work performance 工作绩
效评价

auditor 审核员

authority 权力;权力机构

authorize；delegation 授权;委派

authorized amount 标准总数

authorized strength 编制人员

autocorrelation coefficient 自相关
系数

autocratic leader 专制式领导

automatic call system in emergency
department 急诊自动传呼系统

automatic data processing 自动数据
处理

automatization 自动化

autonomous management 自主管理

autopsy 尸检

auxiliary function 辅助功能

average 平均数

average annual growth rate 平均年
增长率

average attendance per day　平均每日出勤人数

average cost　平均成本

average cost pricing　平均成本定价法

average dose　平均剂量

average elasticity　平均弹性系数

average fixed cost　平均固定成本

average length of hospital stay　平均住院日

average life expectancy　平均预期寿命

average medical expense per inpatient　住院患者人均医疗费用

average medical expense per outpatient　门诊患者人均医疗费用

average number of beds accessible　平均开放病床数

average number of outpatients per day　平均每日门诊人次数

average product of capital　资本平均产量

average product of labour　劳动平均产量

average profit　平均利润

average rate of profit　平均利润率

average revenue　平均收益

average tax rate　平均税率

average total cost　平均总成本

average variable cost　平均可变成本

B

baby boom period　生育高峰

back propagation net-work　误差逆向传播模型

background questions　背景问题

bacteriological laboratory　细菌检验室

balance of manpower　人力平衡

balance of revenue and expenditure　收支平衡

balance sheet　资产负债表

balanced development　均衡发展

balance-sheet approach　平衡表方法

bank loan　银行借款

base hospital　基地医院

base hospital at beachhead　登陆基地医院

base hospital of the front　战区基地医院

base year　基年

baseline comparator　基线比较物

basic faith　基本理念

basic function　基本功能

basic life support　基本生命支持

basic living allowance for laid-off workers　下岗工人基本生活津贴

basic living allowances　基本生活费

basic medical care　基本医疗

basic medical expense insurance　基本医疗费用保险

basic medical insurance system for urban workers　城镇职工基本医疗保险制度

basic medical services　基本医疗服务

basic nursing　基础护理

basic pensions for retirees　离退休人员基本养老金

basic protocol　基本协议

basic quality　基础质量

basic requirements of hospital settings　医院基础条件标准

basic structure　基本结构

basic study　基础研究

basic unit of medical supplies for field first aid　战救药材基数

batch procurement　批量采购

batch production　批量生产

battalion aid station　营救护所

battalion medical post　营卫生所

battle casualties　战斗减员

Bayes' formula　贝叶斯公式

Bayesian method　贝叶斯法

behavior style　行为方式

behavioral pharmacy　行为药学

behavioral science　行为科学

behaviorally anchored rating scales
（BARS）　行为尺度评定量表

benchmark　基准

benchmark of international level
国际水平标准

beneficial cycle　良性循环

beneficiary　受益人

benefit　效益

benefit analysis　效益分析

benefit index of hospital work　医
院工作效益指标

benefit principle　效益原则

benefit-cost ratio　效益-成本比率

best economic batch　最佳经济批量

best evidence　最佳证据

best price　最优价格

bias　偏倚

bid；tender　投标

bidding games　竞标法

bilateral　双向

bilateral arrangement　双边协议

binomial distribution　二项分布

biodiversity　生物多样性

bio-enrichment　生物富集作用

biofeedback　生物反馈

biological half-life　生物半减期

biological marker　生物标志

biomarker of effect　效应标志

biomarker of exposure　暴露生物
标志

biomarker of susceptibility　易感性
生物标志

biomedical model　生物医学模式

biopharmacy　生物药学

bio-psycho-social medical model　生
物-心理-社会医学模式

biostatistics　生物统计学

birth cohort　出生队列

birth rate　出生率

bivariate normal distribution　双变
量正态分布

black box method　黑箱方法

blank control　空白对照

blind method　盲法

blind review　盲态审核

block   区组

block randomization   区组随机化

blood bank   血库

blood donation   献血

blood laboratory   血液实验室

blood product   血液制品

blood security   血液安全

bloodborne disease   血源传播性疾病

Blue Cross   蓝十字

Blue Shield   蓝盾

B-mode ultrasonic room   B超室

board of directors   董事会

body mass index   体重指数

boundary point   边界点

box plot   箱式图

brain death   脑死亡

brain storming   头脑风暴法

branch   分支；分支机构

brand   品牌

bread-and-butter issue   生计问题

break even point   收支相抵点

British Engineering Standards

Associations   英国工程标准协会

bronchoscope room   支气管镜室

buddy aid   互救

budget   预算

budget deficit   预算赤字

budget impact   预算影响

budget line   预算线

budget management   预算管理

budget surplus   预算盈余

building density   建筑密度

burden of disease   疾病负担

burden of proof   举证责任

bureaucracy   官僚主义

burn center   烧伤中心

burning treatment   焚烧处理

business cycle   经济周期

business development   业务拓展

business ethics   商业伦理

business mode   经营方式

business system planning   企业系统
规划

by-product   副产品

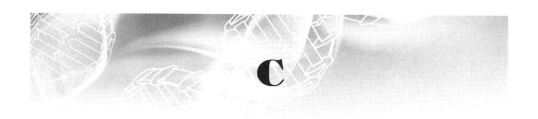

C

campaign rear hospital 战役后方医院

campaign reserve of medical supplies 药材战役储备

Canadian Society for Pharmaceutical Sciences（CSPS） 加拿大药物科学协会

Canadian Standards Association 加拿大标准协会

cancel；revoke；withdraw 吊销

cancer control and prevention center 癌症防治中心

canonical correlation analysis 典型相关分析

canonical correlation coefficient 典型相关系数

canonical correlation variable 典型相关变量

capacity management 能力管理

capital 资本

capital consumption 资本消耗

capital cost 投资成本

capital goods 资本货物

capital injection and system reform 注资改制

capital operation strategy 资本运营战略

capital outlay 资本支出

capital output ratio 资本产出比率

capital principal part 资本主体

capital shortage 资金短缺

capital stock 资本存量

capital transaction 资本交易

capital turnover 资本周转

capitation 按人头付费

carbon monoxide poisoning 一氧化碳中毒

cardiac surgeon 胸外科医师

cardiologist 心血管病医师

carrier 携带者

carry out；implement 贯彻；实施

carry out by actual efforts 身体力行

carry-over effect 残留效应

case 病例

case discussion 病例讨论

case fatality ratio　病死率

case law　案例法

case management　病例管理

case only study　单纯病例研究

case report　病例报告

case review　个案医疗评价

case study　案例分析

case-control study　病例-对照研究

cash analysis　现金分析

cash flow　现金流量

casualties　减员

casualties caused by chemical
　weapons　化学武器减员

casualties caused by conventional
　weapons　常规武器减员

casualties due to diseases　疾病减员

casualties due to noneffectives　卫
　生减员

casualty loss　灾害损失

categorical variable　分类变量

category of diseases　病种

category of wounds　伤类

cause of action　起诉理由

cause-effect relationship　因果联系

cause-specific death rate　死因别死
　亡率

ceiling　最高限额

censored value　截尾值

census　普查

center of disease control　疾病控制
　中心

central disinfection supply room　中
　心消毒供应室

central functional check room　中心
　功能检查室

central hospital　中心医院

central operating room　中心手术室

central tendency　集中趋势

centralization of state power　集权

centralized management　集中管理

centralized procurement　集中采购

centripetal force　向心力

cerebral vascular center　脑血管
　中心

certificate of conformity　合格证书

certificate of quality　质量证书

certification　证书

certification activity　认证活动

certification body　认证机构

Certification Management
　Committee　认证管理委员会

certification quality auditor　认证质
　量审核员

certification quality engineer　认证

质量工程师

certification quality manager   认证质量经理

certification quality technician   认证质量技术员

certification scheme   认证方案

certification system   认证体系

chain hospital   连锁医院

chain-store operations   连锁经营模式

chance nodes   机遇节点

change in demand   需求变化

change in quantity demanded   需求量变化

change in quantity supplied   供给量变化

changing standard   标准转换

channel   渠道

character of hospital culture   医院文化特性

characteristic   特点

characteristic management   特色管理

characteristics   性质

charge   收费

charities   慈善事业

check-and-balance system   制衡机制

chemical burns of eye   化学性眼部灼伤

chemical burns of skin   化学性皮肤灼伤

chemical therapy   化疗

chief head nurse   总护士长

chief information officer   信息主管

chief nurse-master   主任护师

chief of medical branch   医务部主任

chief of medical division   卫生处长

chief of medical section   卫生科长

chief of pharmacy   药局主任

chief pharmacist   主任药师

chief physician   主任医师

chief section member   主任科员

chief technologist   主任技师

chief-deputy physician   副主任医师

children's hospital   儿童医院

China Academy of Traditional Chinese Medicine   中国中医研究院

China Association for Pharmaceutical Equipment （CAPE）   中国制药装备行业协会

China Association of Chinese Medicine   中华中医药学会

China Insurance Regulatory
　　Commission　中国保监会

China Nonprescription Medicines
　　Association（CNMA）　中国非处方
　　药物协会

China Pharmaceutical Packaging
　　Association　中国医药包装协会

China Quality Certification Center
　　for Medical Devices　中国医疗器
　　械质量认证中心

Chinese drugs pharmacist in charge
　　主管中药师

Chinese medicine　中医药

Chinese medicine pharmacist　中
　　药师

Chinese medicine pharmacy　中药房

Chinese medicine preparation
　　laboratory　中药制剂室

Chinese Pharmaceutical Association
　　中国药学会

Chinese Pharmacopoeia　中国药典

chi-square distribution　卡方分布

chi-square test　卡方检验

chronic obstructive pulmonary
　　disease（COPD）　慢性阻塞性肺
　　疾病

chronic respiratory disease

questionnaire（RDQ）　慢性呼吸疾
　　病问卷

circle quality control　循环质量控制

citation bias　引用偏倚

civil defense rescue station　民防救
　　护站

civil law　大陆法；民法

civil lawsuit　民事诉讼

civil procedure law　民事诉讼法

civil right　民事权利

civil right act　人权法案

civilian；civil affairs　民事

claim　保险索赔

claim rejected　拒赔

claim right　索取权

claims data　申报资料

classical economics　古典经济学

classification　分类

classification of diseases　疾病分类

Classification of International
　　Standard　国际标准分类

clause　条款

cleanness section　清洁区

clinic medical quality　临床医疗质量

clinical audit　临床审计

clinical decision analysis　临床决策
　　分析

clinical department　临床科室

clinical economics　临床经济学

clinical epidemiology　临床流行病学

clinical evaluation　临床评价

clinical evidence　临床证据

clinical guideline　临床指南

clinical information system　临床信
　息系统

clinical nursing conductor　临床护理
　指挥

clinical outcome　临床结局

clinical path（CP）临床路径

clinical pharmacodynamics　临床药
　效学

clinical pharmacology　临床药理学

clinical pharmacology base　临床药
　理基地

clinical pharmacy　临床药学

clinical practice guideline　临床实践
　指南

clinical professor　临床教授

clinical psychology　临床心理学

clinical regulations　临床规章制度

clinical research evidence　临床研究
　证据

clinical skills and competence　临床
　技能

clinical trial　临床试验

clinician　临床医师

closed economy　封闭经济

clothing supply management　被服
　供应管理

cluster analysis　聚类分析

cluster index　聚集指数

cluster sampling　整群抽样

Cobb-Douglas　柯布-道格拉斯

Cobb-Douglas production function
　柯布-道格拉斯生产函数

Cochrane collaboration network　科
　克伦协作网

Cochrane library　科克伦图书馆

Cochrane systematic review　科克伦
　系统评价

code of medical equipment　医疗设
　备代码

co-defendant　共同被告

codification　法律汇编

coefficient of determination　决定
　系数

coefficient of kurtosis　峰度系数

coefficient of regression　回归系数

coefficient of skewness　偏度系数

coefficient of variation　变异系数

cognition　认知

cognitive dissonance　认知失调

cognitive process　认知过程

cognitive psychology　认知心理学

cognitive skill　认知技能

cognitive structure　认知结构

cognitive style　认知方式

coherent system　协调系统

cohesion　凝聚力

cohort　队列

cohort effect　队列效应

cohort life table　队列寿命表

cohort study　队列研究

co-insurance　共负保险

collective capital　集体资本

collective ownership　集体所有

collective shares　集体股

collective thinking　集体思维

collectivism　集体主义

collectivity power　集体力量

collocation room　配置室

color ultrasonic room　彩超室

combat readiness storage　战备储备

combat support hospital　战斗支援
　医院

combat zone　作战区

combat zone hospital　前沿兵站医院

combination　组合化

combined Chinese and western
　medicine　中西医结合

combined weight　组合权重

combined/pooled variance　合并
　方差

combining site　结合点

come into force　生效

command　命令；指挥

command and control of health
　service　卫勤组织指挥

command economy　命令经济

commercial insurance　商业保险

commercial medical insurance　商业
　医疗保险

commercial value　商业价值

commercialization　商品化

commissar　政委

commission　回扣

Commission on Macroeconomics and
　Health　宏观经济与健康委员会

commission on the accreditation for
　hospital　医院评审委员会

committee draft　委员会草案

committee office　委员会办公室

committee on certification　认证委
　员会

committee on conformity assessment

合格评定委员会

commodity   商品

commodity combination   商品组合

commodity market   商品市场

commodity space   商品空间

common disease   常见病

common law   普通法;习惯法

common needs of the society   社会
公共需要

common property   公用财产

common regression coefficient   公
共回归系数

common vision   共同愿景

commonality health equipment   公
共卫生设备

commonweal   公益性

communication   沟通;通信

communication management   通信
管理

community   社区

community financing   社区筹资

community health care center   社区
保健中心

community health education(CHE)
社区卫生教育

community health service institutions
社区卫生服务机构

community health service(CHS)   社
区卫生服务

community health workers(CHW)
社区卫生工作者

community hospital   社区医院

community long-term nursing   社区
长期护理

community medical care   社区医疗

community medicine   社区医学

community nurse   社区护士

community nursing home   社区老年
护理服务机构

community practitioner   社区医生

Community Sanitation Department
社区卫生司

community service   社区服务

community-based rehabilitation   社
区康复服务

company medical room   连卫生室

comparative advantage   比较优势

comparision price system   比较定价

compensable transfer; remunerative
transfer   有偿转让

compensated demand function   补偿
需求函数

compensating variation in income
收入补偿变量

compensation　赔偿

compensation of medical cost　医疗
费用赔偿

compensation pay-outs　保险赔付
金额

compensation principles　补偿原则

competence　能力

competing risk　竞争风险

competition　竞争

competition strategy　竞争战略

competitive advantage　竞争性优势

competitive appointment system　竞
争聘任制度

competitive decision making；decision
under conflict　竞争型决策

competitive market　竞争性市场

competitive principle　竞争性原则

competitive procurement　竞争采购

competitiveness resources　竞争力
资源

complement each other　优势互补

complement goods　互补品

complete cost　完全成本

complete information　完全信息

complete life table　完全寿命表

complete randomization　完全随
机化

completely random design　完全随
机设计

completeness　完备性

complex　复合性

compliance　依从性

comply　履行

compound Poisson　复合泊松

comprehensive evaluating method
综合评价法

comprehensive evaluation　综合评比

comprehensive forecasting　综合
预测

comprehensive hospital　综合医院

comprehensive index　综合指标

comprehensive management system
综合管理体系

comprehensive quality　综合素质

comprehensiveness　综合性

compulsory　强制性

compulsory certificate　强制性认证

compulsory insurance　强制保险（义
务保险）

compulsory；obligative　强制

computer aided software engineering
计算机辅助软件工程

computer equipment　计算机装备

computerized management　计算机

管理

computerized management of
medical records   病案计算机管理

computerized simulation method   计
算机模拟法

concept system   概念系统

concordant   协调性

concurrent validity   同期效度

condition for efficiency in
production   生产的最优条件

conditional logistic regression   条件
逻辑斯谛回归

conditional variance   条件方差

conditioned reflex（CR）   条件反射

confidence   自信

confidence interval   可信区间

confidence limit   可信限

configuration   配置

confirmatory factor analysis   证实
性因子分析

confirmatory study   验证性研究

confirmed rate within three days
三日确诊率

confiscate   没收

conflict   冲突

conflict of interests   利益冲突

conform requirements   符合要求

conformity assessment   合格评定

conformity certification   合格认证

conformity certification   质量认证

conformity testing   合格测试

confounder   混杂因子

confounding   混杂

confounding bias   混杂偏倚

confounding factor   混杂因素

conjoint analysis   联合分析

connotation   内涵

consciousness   意识

consciousness of responsibility   责
任感

consensus   一致

consent   同意

consistency   一致性

consistency of the association   关联
的一致性

consistency rate of diagnosis   诊断
符合率

consolidated health care systems   卫
生保健系统

constancy assumption   稳定性假设

constant return to scale   规模收益
不变

constituent ratio of all kind of staffs
in hospital   医院人员构成比

constituent ratio of all kinds of health and technical staff in hospital　医院卫生技术人员构成比

constituent ratio of disease　疾病构成比

Constitution of the People's Republic of China　中华人民共和国宪法

constraint force　约束力

construct validity　结构效度

construction of hospital culture　医院文化构建

consultation　会诊

consulting room　诊室

consumer　消费者

consumer behavior　消费者行为

consumer choice　消费者选择

consumer equilibrium　消费者均衡

consumer optimization　消费者优化

consumer preference　消费者偏好

consumer psychology　消费心理学

consumer surplus　消费者剩余

consumer theory　消费者理论

consumer's budget line　消费者预算线

consumption　消费

consumption combination　消费组合

consumption possibility　消费可能

consumption quota of medical supplies　药材消耗限额

consumption space　消费空间

contagion　传染

contemporary management system　现代管理制度

content validity　内容效度

contingency rule；strain criteria　应变准则

contingency strategy　应变策略

contingency theory　权变理论

contingent evaluation（CV）　条件评估

continuous education　继续教育

continuous function　连续函数

continuous improvement　持续改进

continuous improvement of the organization　组织持续改进

continuous medical education　继续医学教育

continuous quality improvement　持续质量改进

continuous variable　连续性变量

contraceptive prevalence rate　节育率（避孕率）

contract　合同

contract curve　契约曲线

contracted physician　合同制医师

contractual operation　承包经营

contrast　对比

contravene a law　违法

contributor　出资人;捐助者

control　控制

control chart　控制图

control methods　控制手段

control object　控制对象

control of medical cost　医院费用
控制

control point of medical quality　医
疗质量控制点

control procedure for customer
property　顾客财产控制程序

control process　控制过程

control right　控制权

control standard of medical quality
医疗质量控制标准

control system of medical quality
医疗质量控制系统

control technology　控制技术

control unit　控制单位

control variable　控制变量

controllable cost　可控成本

controllable input　可控输入

controlled clinical trial　临床对照
试验

convalescence hospital　康复医院

convenience sampling　便利抽样

conventional hospital　传统型医院

convergence competition　趋同竞争

convergent validity　平行效度

cooking equipment　炊事设备

cooperate pooling model　合作联营
模式

cooperative health service　合作
医疗

cooperative medical system　合作医
疗制度

coordinated development　协调发展

coordination　协调

coordination of health service
institutions　卫勤协同

co-payment　共同分摊费用

core competency　关键才能

core competitiveness　核心竞争力

core employee　核心员工

core grade　核心职系

core journal　核心期刊

core leader　核心领导

core value　核心价值

corporate governance structure　法

人治理结构

corporate plan   整体计划

corporeal right   占有权

correction   校正

correction factor   修正因子

corrective action   纠正措施

correlation analysis   相关性分析

correlation coefficient   相关系数

correlation index   相关指数

correlation matrix   相关矩阵

correlative analysis method   相关分
析法

cost accounting   成本核算

cost analysis   成本分析

cost benefit analysis   成本-效益分析

cost benefit ratio   成本-效益比率

cost budget   成本预算

cost center   成本中心

cost competitiveness   成本竞争力

cost consciousness   费用意识

cost consequence analysis   成本结果
分析

cost-effectiveness analysis   成本-效
果分析

cost effectiveness ratio   成本效果
比率

cost efficiency   成本效率

cost function   成本函数

cost minimization   成本最小化

cost minimization analysis   最小成
本分析

cost of goods sold   销货成本

cost of illness   疾病成本

cost of lost time   时间损失成本

cost of therapy   疾病治疗成本

cost utility analysis   成本-效用分析

cost utility ratio   成本-效用比率

cost-benefit analysis   成本-效益分析

cost-effectiveness   成本效果

cost-effectiveness analysis   成本-效
果分析

cost-sharing   费用分担

cost-volume-profit analysis   本量利
分析

council   理事会

Council of Medical Sciences and
Technology   医学科学技术委员会

counselor；mentor   辅导者

counterclaim   反诉

countermeasure   对策

court   法院

court of common pleas   民诉法院

court of second instance   二审法院

covariate   协变量

coverage   保险总额,覆盖

coverage rate   覆盖率

Cox proportional hazard model   考
克斯比例风险模型

creative thinking   创造性思维

credibility   可信度

credibility factor   信度因子

credit   信用

credit and reputation   信誉

credit insurance   信用保险

creditor   债权人

criminal law   刑法

criminal procedure law   刑事诉讼法

criminal responsibility   刑事责任

crisis public relations   危机公关

criterion research   规范研究

criterion validity   标准效度

criterion-related validity   准则效度

critical appraisal   严格评价

critical control point   关键控制点

critical incident method   关键事
件法

critical stock position   存货短缺

critical value   临界值

cross elasticity of demand   需求的
交叉弹性

cross infection   交叉感染

cross integration   交叉融合

cross-culture propagation   跨文化
传播

cross-over design   交叉设计

cross-over experiment   交叉试验

cross-sectional study   横断面研究

cross-subsidy   交叉补助

crude birth rate   粗出生率

crude death rate   粗死亡率

crude incidence rate   粗发病率

cultural atmosphere   文化氛围

culture   文化

cumulative death rate   累计死亡率

cumulative failure rate   累计失败率

cumulative incidence rate   累计发
病率

cure   治愈

cure rate   治愈率

currency capital   货币资本

current account with others   往来
账户

current assets   流动资产

current liabilities   流动负债

current life table   现时寿命表

curve fitting   曲线拟合

customer   顾客

customer communication   顾客沟通

customer complaint   顾客投诉

customer feedback   顾客反馈

customer oriented   顾客导向

customer property   顾客财产

customer relationship management
　　客户关系管理

customer satisfaction   顾客满意

customer service   顾客服务

customer service contact form   顾客
　　服务联系表

customer's value chain   顾客价值链

cybernetics   控制论

cycle length   周期时间

cystoscopy room   膀胱镜室

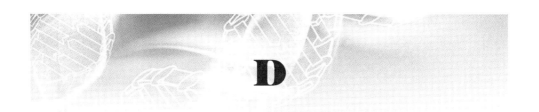

D

daily average casualties　平均减员

daily care of a patient　患者的日常护理

daily service management　日常服务管理

damage；harm；hazard；injury　损伤

data backup　数据备分

data collection　资料收集

data management　数据管理

data mining　数据挖掘

data photocopy　资料复印

data warehouse　数据仓库

database　数据库

database management system　数据库管理系统

database system　数据库系统

day care hospital　日间医院

De Bike Rules　德比克法则

deal cost；sanction cost　交易成本

dealing flux　交易流量

debt　负债

decease；death；die　死亡

decentralization　分权

decision　决策

decision analysis　决策分析

decision goal　决策目标

decision model　决策模式

decision rule　决策原则

decision science　决策科学

decision support system　决策支持系统

decision technique　决策技术

decision theory　决策论

decision tree　决策树

decision tree analysis　决策树分析

decision under risk　风险型决策

decision under uncertainty　非确定型决策

decision-making layer　决策层

decision-making process　决策过程

decision-making study　决策学

decisive action　决定作用

decode　译码

decompression sickness　减压病

decontamination group　洗消组

decreasing return to scale   规模收益
递减

decree   法令

deductible   起付线(免赔额)

deduction   演绎法

defective product   次品

defendant   被告

deferred variable cost   延期变动
成本

definitive treatment   确定性治疗

deformity；disability   残疾

degree of freedom（DF）   自由度

delay to diagnose and treat   延误
诊疗

delayed report   迟报

delivery mortality in hospital   院内
分娩死亡率

delivery room   产房

Delphi method   德尔菲方法；专家咨
询法

demand   需求

demand analysis   需求分析

demand curve   需求曲线

demand cycle   需求周期

demand elasticity   需求弹性

demand function   需求函数

demand management   需求管理

demand price   需求价格

demand schedule   需求表

demobilized armymen   复员转业
军人

democratic leader   民主式领导

demographic factor   人口因素

dentist   牙科医师

dentistry   牙科学

department   部门

department chief   科室主任

department of anesthesiology   麻
醉科

department of anus & intestine
surgery   肛肠外科

department of bone fracture   骨
伤科

department of burn surgery   烧伤科

department of cardiac surgery   心脏
外科

department of cardiology   心脏病科

department of cerebral surgery   脑
外科

department of chemotherapy   化
疗科

department of dentistry   牙科

department of dermatology   皮肤科

department of drug selling   药品销

售部门

department of emergency　急诊科

department of endocrinology　内分泌科

department of gastroenterology　消化科

department of general surgery　普外科

department of geriatrics　老年科

department of health care　保健科

department of health care and prevention　预防保健科

Department of Health Regulation and Supervision　卫生法制与监督司

department of health service research　卫勤医学研究室

department of hematology　血液科

department of hepatobiliary surgery　肝胆外科

department of infection　传染科

department of internal medicine　内科

department of laboratory　检验科

department of medical administration　医政司

department of medical records　病

案室

department of nephrology　肾内科

department of neurology　神经内科

department of neurosurgery　神经外科

department of nuclear medicine　核医学科

department of oncology　肿瘤科

department of ophthalmology　眼科

department of orthopedics　矫形外科

department of otorhinolaryngology　耳鼻喉科

department of out-patient　门诊部

department of pathology　病理科

department of pediatric surgery　儿童外科

department of pediatrics　儿科

department of personnel　人事司

department of pharmacology　药理科

department of pharmacy　药学部

department of plastic surgery　整形外科

department of psychiatry　精神病科

department of purchasing　采购部门

department of radiation　放射科

department of radiotherapy　放疗科

department of respiratory medicine
　呼吸科

department of rheumatology　风
　湿科

Department of Science，Technology
　and Education　科技教育司

department of special treatment　特
　诊科

department of sport medicine　运动
　医学科

department of stomatology　口腔科

department of surgery　外科

department of thoracic surgery　胸
　外科

department of traditional Chinese
　medicine　中医科

department of traumatology　创伤
　外科

department of ultrasonography　超
　声科

department of urology　泌尿科

department of venereology　性病科

departmental cost accounting　科室
　成本核算

departments of medical care　医疗
　科室

dependent variable　应变量

deployment of health service units
　卫勤机构配置

deposit premium　预付保险费

depot of medical materials　药材
　仓库

depreciation　折旧

deputy chief head nurse　副总护
　士长

deputy chief section member　副主
　任科员

deputy director general　副处长

deputy director of hospital　医院副
　院长

deputy section chief　副科长

deputy section director　科副主任

deputy supervisor of nursing care
　副护士长

dereliction of duty　玩忽职守

derivative　导数

derivative policy　派生政策

derive demand　派生需求

dermatologist　皮肤科医师

dermatology　皮肤学

descending cost　成本递减

descending returns to scale　规模报
　酬递减

descriptive study　描述性研究

destroy；ruin　销毁

determinant factor，decisive factor　决定因素

determination of hospital beds　病床编设

deterministic model　确定性模型

development opportunity　发展机会

development plan　发展计划

development target　发展目标

developmental strategy　发展战略

deviation　偏差

deviation degree　偏离程度

diagnosis　诊断

diagnosis bias　诊断偏倚

diagnosis related groups（DRG）　诊断相关组

diagnostic equipment　诊断设备

diagnostic fee　诊察费

diagnostic related groups（DRGs）　按疾病诊断分类支付

diagnostic-therapeutic cycle　诊断治疗周期

died of wounds　伤死

diet fee　伙食费

differentiate　分化

differentiated pricing　区别定价

differentiation strategy　差异化战略

digital signal processor　数字信号处理器

digital subtraction angiography　数字减影血管造影技术

diminishing marginal substitution　边际替代递减

diminishing marginal utility　边际效用递减

diminishing return　收益递减

direct application of international standard　国际标准的直接应用

direct benefit　直接效益

direct burden　直接经济负担

direct cost　直接成本

direct financing　直接融资

direct investment　直接投资

direct labor　直接人工

directional plans　方向性计划

director of hospital　医院院长

director of medical department　医政司长

director of nursing department　护理部主任

director of outpatient department　门诊部主任

director of pharmacy store　药库

主任

director of political department 政治部(处)主任

director of the internal medicine department 内科主任

director of the surgical department 外科主任

directorate 董事会

director's office 主任办公室

disability adjusted life years 失能调整生命年

disabled person 残疾人

disadvantaged groups 弱势群体

disaster backup 灾难备份

disaster management 灾备管理

disaster medicine 灾害医学

disaster preparedness 灾备

disaster preparedness training 灾备训练

disaster recovery 灾难恢复

discharge 出院

discipline 学科

discipline resources 学科资源

discipline technology resources 学科技术资源

discomfort;disorder 不适

discount 折扣;贴现

discount rate 贴现率

discrete distribution 离散型分布

discrete property 分立的产权

discrete type 离散型

discrete variable 离散变量

discretion 离散度

discriminant analysis 判别分析

disease 疾病

disease causation 疾病因果关系

Disease Defense and Command Office 疾病预防控制局

disease monitoring 疾病监测

disease specific instruments 疾病专用量表

disease-based cost accounting 病种医疗成本核算

disease-based model 基于疾病的模型

disease-related quality control 单病种质量控制

disequilibrium 非均衡

disinfection 消毒

disinfection isolation 消毒隔离

disorder 无序

disordered competition 无序竞争

disposable income per capita in urban areas 城镇居民人均可支配

收入

disposition district of aid station 救护所配置地域

disposition right 处置权

disposition；layout 布局

dispute 争议

disruption of hospital culture 医院文化的衰败

distribution according to asset 按资分配

distribution according to knowledge 按知分配

distribution according to work 按劳分配

distribution function 分布函数

distribution of benefits 利益分布

distribution of disease 疾病分布

distribution of medical supplies 药材分配

distribution standard 配置标准

distribution theory of marginal productivity 边际生产率分配理论

district court 地方法院

diverse forms of ownership 多种所有制

diversification of forms 形式多样化

diversification of investment 投资渠道多元化

diversity jurisdiction 多元管辖权

diversity；multiplicity；variety；versatility 多样性

dividend 股息

dividends income 股利收入

division chief 处长

division of health service 卫勤处

division of medical supplies 药材处

division of medical treatment 医疗处

dizzy wheel effect 晕轮效应

doctor of traditional Chinese medicine 中医师

doctor；physician 内科医师

doctor-in-charge 主治医师

doctor-patient relationship 医患关系

doctor's office 医师办公室

doctor's workshop 医师工作间

document 文书档案

document management 文件档案管理

documents for medical evacuation 医疗后送文件袋

dominance 显性

dominated therapy　劣势治疗

dose effect　剂量效应

dose-effect curve　剂量-效应曲线

dose-response relationship　剂量-反应关系

dose-survival curve　剂量-存活曲线

double blind method　双盲法

double blinded trial　双盲试验

double counting　双重计算

double dissociation　双重分离

double entry　双份录入

double estimation　双重估计

double sampling　二次抽样

double stimulation　双模拟

double test method　二次检测法

double-blind and double-dummy technique　双盲双模拟技术

downsize staffs and improve efficiency　减员增效

draft　草案

dressing bowl　换药碗

driving right　主动权

drug　药品

drug administration　药政管理

drug analysis　药物分析

drug batch number　药品批号

drug expenditure　药品支出

drug expenditure per capita　人均药品费用

drug inspector　药品监督员

drug management method　药品管理办法

drug operation　药品经营

drug price　药品价格

drug quality control　药品质量监督

drug quality management　药品质量管理

drug quality standard　药品质量标准

drug resistance；drug tolerance　耐药性

drug safety　药品安全

drug substance　原料药

drug use evaluation　药物利用度评估

drug utilization　药物利用

drug utilization index　药物利用指数

DSA room　心导管室

dual structure of authority　双重权力结构

duality　二重性

due process　正当程序

dummy variables　哑变量

durable goods　耐用品

duration of insurance　保险期

duty　职务

duty evaluation　职务评审

dynamic analysis　动态分析

dynamic combination　动态组合

dynamic management　动态管理

dynamic model　动态模型

dynamic monitoring　动态监测

dynamic population　动态人群

dynamic programming　动态规划

dysfunction of pharmaceutical
　market　药品市场失灵

E

early treatment　早期治疗

early-warning system　预警机制

ear-nose-throat doctor　耳鼻喉科
　医师

echocardiography room　超声心动
　图室

ecological construction　生态建筑

ecological environment　生态环境

ecological epidemiology　生态流行
　病学

ecological medical model　生态医学
　模式

ecology comparison study　生态比较
　研究

ecology study　生态研究

ecology trend study　生态趋势研究

econometric model analysis　计量模
　型分析

econometrics　计量经济学

economic analysis　经济学分析

economic benefit　经济效益

economic cost　经济成本

economic decision　经济决策

economic efficiency　经济效率

economic evaluation　经济学评价

economic model　经济模型

economic order quantity　经济定货
　量法

economic outcomes　经济学结果

economic prediction　经营预测

economic profit　经济利润

economic regulation　经济法规

economic rent　经济租金

economic restructuring　经济结构
　调整

economic scale　经济规模

economic system　经济体系

economic welfare　经济福利

economics　经济学

economy　经济

economy of scale　规模经济

ecosystem　生态系统

ecosystem disequilibrium　生态失衡

editing committee　编辑委员会

education and research　教学科研

education and training　教育培训

educational rehabilitation　教育康复

effect magnitude　效应尺度

effect of medicine　药物效果

effect size　效应量

effective allocation　有效配置

effective communication　有效沟通

effective management　有效管理

effective presentation　有效表达

effectiveness　效果

efficacy　效能

efficiency　效率

efficiency of experiment　实验效率

efficiency parameter　效率参数

efficiency wage　效率工资

efficient scale　有效规模

ego-defense　自我防御

E-health　电子健康

eigenvalue　特征值

elasticity　弹性

elasticity of substitution　替代弹性

elasticity rule　弹性法则

electrocardiogram room　心电图室

electromyogram room　肌电图室

electronic commerce　电子商务

electronic data interchange　电子数
据交换

electronic government　电子政务

electronic medical record　电子病历

elements of medical quality　医疗质
量要素

elements of medical system　医疗系
统构件

emergency　急诊

emergency care　急救

emergency center　急救中心

emergency disease spectrum　急诊疾
病谱

emergency duty room　急诊值班室

emergency events　突发事件

emergency fee　急诊费

emergency first-visit responsibility
system　急诊首诊负责制

emergency institutionalized
management　急诊制度化管理

emergency intensive care unit　急诊
监护室

emergency internal medicine
department　急诊内科

emergency laboratory　急诊化验室

emergency measure　紧急措施

emergency medical care　紧急救治

emergency medical care information
system　急救医疗信息系统

emergency medical care system　急

救医疗系统

emergency medical management model 急救医疗管理模式

emergency mobile hospital 应急机动医院

emergency observation room 急诊观察室

emergency obstetrics and gynecology department 急诊妇产科

emergency operation room 急诊手术室

emergency pediatrics department 急诊儿科

emergency pharmacy 急诊药房

emergency programmed management 急诊程序化管理

emergency registration & cashier office 急诊收费挂号

emergency room 急诊室

emergency service；first aid station （FAP） 急救站

emergency standardization management 急诊标准化管理

emergency surgery department 急诊外科

emergency therapeutic room 急诊治疗室

emergency-response management 应急管理

empirical approach 经验法

empirical medicine 经验医学

employee 雇员

employee benefits 职工福利

employee education 职工教育

employer 雇主

employment 就业

employment system 劳动用工制度

employment（work）injury insurance 工伤保险

encoding 编码

encouragement system 奖励制度

end point 观察终点

endemic 地方病

endocrinology 内分泌学

endogenous fund 内源性资金

endogenous health resources 内生性卫生资源

endogenous hospital infection 内源性医院感染

endogenous medical resources 内生性医疗资源

endogenous variable 内生变量

endoscopy room 内镜室

endowment insurance 养老保险

end-stage renal disease（ESRD）　终
末期肾病

engaging system　聘用制

Engel curve　恩格尔曲线

engineer　工程师；工程技术人员

enteroscopy room　肠镜室

enterprise interest　企业利益

enterprise resources planning　企业
资源计划

entity　实体

entity-relationship model　实体关系
模型

entry barriers　进入壁垒

enumeration data　计数资料

environment beautification　环境
美化

environment variable　环境变量

environment virescence　环境绿化

environmental audit　环境审核

environmental hygiene　环境卫生学

environmental management system
环境管理体系

environmental monitoring　环境
监测

environmental pollution　环境污染

environmental protection　环境保护

epidemic　流行病

epidemic prevention　卫生防疫

epidemic prevention station　防疫站

epidemic situation　疫情

epidemic situation monitoring　疫情
监测

epidemiology　流行病学

epidemiology in hospital infection
医院感染流行病学

equal competition　公平竞争

equal right　同等权利

equal treatment　平等待遇

equilibrium　均衡

equilibrium condition　均衡条件

equilibrium price　均衡价格

equilibrium quantity　均衡产量

equipment　设备

equipment control procedure　设备
控制程序

equipment maintenance　设备维修

equipment management　设备管理

equipment well-used rate　设备完
好率

equity　公平性

equity adjustments　权益调整

equity in health　健康公平性

equivalence　等效

equivalent variation in income　收

入等价变量

ergonomics 工效学

error 误差

error check mechanism 纠错机制

essence of insurance 保险要素

essential drugs 基本药品

essential health care services 基本卫生服务

essential medical service 基本医疗服务

establishment of quality index 质量指标构建

esteem needs 尊敬的需要

estimate 评价

estimating the cost of illness 疾病成本估计

estimation 估计

estimation of bed requirements 床位需求量估算

estimation of health service transport 卫勤运力预计

estimation of parameter 参数估计

estimation of requirement of medical supplies 药材预算

ethics 伦理

etiologic fraction 病因分值

eugenics 优生优育

European Committee for Standardization 欧洲标准化委员会

European Federation for Medical Informatics 医学信息学欧洲联盟

European Foundation for Quality Management 欧洲质量管理基金

European Quality Award 欧洲质量奖

EuroQol 5-Dimensions（EQ-5D） 欧洲五维生存质量量表

euthanasia 安乐死

evacuation document envelope 后送文件袋

evacuation hospital 后送医院

evacuation triage 后送分类

evaluation 评价

evaluation and measurement 评估测量

evaluation grade 评价等级

evaluation index 评价指标

evaluation method 评价方法

evaluation model 评价模型

evaluation of human resources 人力资源评估

evaluation standard 评价标准

event pathway 事件路径

evidence-based decision-making　循证决策

evidence-based diagnosis　循证诊断

evidence-based gynecology & obstetrics　循证妇产科学

evidence-based health care　循证卫生保健

evidence-based internal medicine　循证内科学

evidence-based medical education　循证医学教育

evidence-based medical resources　循证医学资源

evidence-based medical standard　循证医学标准

evidence-based medicine　循证医学

evidence-based nursing　循证护理

evidence-based pediatrics　循证儿科学

evidence-based selection　循证筛选

evidence-based surgery　循证外科学

examination & therapeutic room　检查治疗室

examination by letter　函审

examination room　检查室

examination system for doctors' qualification　医师资格考试制度

examination system for pharmacists' qualification　药师资格考试制度

examine and approve　审批

excess of loss coverage　超额赔款保险

excess profit　超额利润

excess-capacity theorem　过度生产能力定理

exclusion　排斥性；排他性

exclusion criteria　排除标准

execution level　执行层

exemption　豁免

exogenous health resources　外源性卫生资源

exogenous hospital infection　外源性医院感染

exogenous medical resources　外源性医疗资源

exogenous variables　外生变量

expansion　扩展性

expectation　期望

expected objective　预期目标

expected utility　期望效用

expected value　期望值

expected value principle　期望值原理

expense management　费用管理

experiment control　实验对照

experiment design　实验设计

experiment effect　实验效应

experiment object　实验对象

experiment study　实验研究

experiment study design　实验研究
　设计

experimental fact　经验事实

experimental method　实验法

expert consultation　专家咨询

expert forecasting　专家预测

explicit cost　显性成本

exploratory forecasting　探索性预测

exponential　指数

exponential claim amounts　指数索
　赔量

exponential principle　指数原理

exponential smoothing method　指
　数平滑法

export control　出口管理

export license control　出口许可证
　制度

exposure　暴露

extensive development model　粗放
　型发展模式

extensive management　粗放管理

external benefit　外部收益;外部
　效益

external cost　外部成本

external economy　外部经济

external environment　外部环境

external factor　外部因素

external supervision　外部监督

externality　外延性

extraneous factor　外来因素

extrapolation models　外推模型

extreme value　极端值

F

face to face interview　面对面访问

face validity　表面效度

factor analysis　因子分析

factor demand　需求要素

factor evaluation　因素评价法

factor of insurance　保险因子

factor substitution　替代要素

factor supply　供给要素

factorial design　析因设计

factorial experiment　析因试验

factorial experiment design　析因试
　验设计

factual input to the project　项目实
　际投入额

failure event　失效事件

fairness；equity　公平性

fairness in financial contribution
　费用分担的公平性

fairness of financial contribution
　筹资的公平性

false negative rate　假阴性率；漏
　诊率

false positive rate　假阳性率；误诊率

familial aggregation　家族(庭)聚
　集性

familial aggregation study　家族
　(庭)聚集性研究

family-based rehabilitation　家庭
　康复

family doctor　家庭医师

family hospital　家属医院

family planning　计划生育

family resemblance　家族(庭)相
　似性

family sick-beds　家庭病床

family-style nursing　家庭化护理

feasibility　可行性

feasibility of measurement　测量的
　可行性

feasibility research　可行性研究

featured discipline　特色专科

feedback　反馈

feedback control　反馈控制

feedback frequency　反馈频率

feedback gain　反馈强度

fee-for-service　按服务付费

fetal monitor room　胎心监护室

fibrescope room　纤维镜室

field　野战

field aid station　野战医疗所

field blood transfusion　野战输血

field control　现场控制

field hospital　野战医院

field hospital for infectious diseases　野战传染病医院

field hospital for lightly wounded　野战轻伤病医院

field hospital for war gas-injury　野战毒剂伤医院

field medical history　野战病历

field medical team　野战医疗队

field operation room　野战手术室

field trial　现场试验

final accounts　决算

final goods　最终产品

finance　财务

Finance and Economy Committee　财政经济委员会

finance asset　金融资产

financial account of cost　成本决算

financial accounting　财务会计

financial activities　财务活动

financial affairs department　财务科

financial analysis　财务分析

financial assets　财务资本

financial capacity　财政承受能力

financial capital　金融资本

financial capital management　金融资本运营

financial control　财务控制

financial entity　财务实体

financial expenditure　财政支出

financial forecast　财务预测

financial impact　财务影响

financial index　财务指标

financial management　财政管理

financial management environment　财务管理环境

financial management objectives　财务管理目标

financial planning　财务计划

financial policy　财务政策

financial regulations　财务制度

financial revenue　财政收入

financial risk　财务风险

financial situation of hospital　医院财务状况

financial subsidy　财政补助

financial supervision　财务监督

financing　投融资策略

fine for delaying payment　滞纳金

finite population　有限总体

finite population correction factor
　有限总体校正因子

first aid　急救

first aid in frontline　火线抢救

first encounter　首诊

first hearing；first review　初审

first line hospital　一线医院

first party inspection　第一方检验

first-class hospital at grade 1　一级
　甲等医院

first-class hospital at grade 2　二级
　甲等医院

first-class hospital at grade 3　三级
　甲等医院

fit and unfit level　优劣程度

fitting of distribution　分布拟合

five techniques of first aid　战救 5
　项技术

fixed assets　固定资产

fixed capital　固定资本

fixed cohort　固定队列

fixed cost　固定成本

fixed effect　固定效应

fixed effect model　固定效应模型

fixed information　固定信息

fixed input　固定投入

fixed order quantity　固定批量法

fixed premium　固定保费

flaw analysis　缺陷分析

flexibility　柔性

flexible system　柔性系统

floating population　流动人口

Flood Control Act　《水灾控制法案》

fluoroscopy　透视室

focus group discussion　专题小组
　讨论

follow-up　随访

follow-up prevalence study　随访患
　病率研究

food additives　食物添加剂

food and drink permit　食品及饮品
　许可证

Food and Drug Administration
　（FDA）　食品药品监督管理局

food hygiene law　食品卫生法

food hygiene；food sanitation　食品
　卫生

food poisoning　食物中毒

food-borne disease　因食物而引起的
　疾病

food-borne infection and intoxication
　因食物而引起的感染与中毒

forecast science　预测学

forecasting procedure　预测程序

foreground questions　前景问题

forensic appraisal　司法鉴定

forensic medicine　法医学

forest plots　森林图

form of medical system　医疗系统组成

form of periodical payments　定期支付形式

formal organization　正式组织

formal planning　正式计划

formulary　医院用药目录

for-profit organization　营利性组织

forward design　前向设计

four administration points　四定

fourfold table　四格表

free entry　自由进入

free medical service　免费医疗

free use　无偿使用

freedom of choice　自由选择

frequency distribution　频数分布

frequency table　频数分布表

frequently encountered disease　多发病

friction cost　摩擦成本

Friedman test　弗里德曼检验

front edge　前沿

frontier branches of science　边缘学科

full cost　完全成本

full credibility for claim numbers　索赔的完全信度

function of hospital performance assessment　医院绩效评估

functional analysis　功能分析

functional department　职能科室

functional disturbance；functional impairment　功能障碍

functional living index-cancer（FLIC）　癌症患者生活功能指数

functional value method　功能价值法

fund in individual medical insurance account　个人医疗账户基金

fund management　资金管理

fundamental ability　基本能力

fundamental analysis　基本分析

fundamental principles of medical management　医疗管理基本原则

fundamental rights　基本权利

fundamental principle　基本原则

funding system　基金式

funds　基金

funds for military medical service
军队卫生事业费

funds of basic medical insurance 基本医疗保险基金

funds of insurance 保险基金

funds of medical insurance 医疗保险基金

funds raised by oneself 自筹资金

future value 未来值

fuzzy clustering analysis 模糊聚类分析

fuzzy comprehensive assessment 模糊综合评价

fuzzy mathematics 模糊数学

fuzzy matrix 模糊矩阵

fuzzy model 模糊模型

fuzzy set 模糊集

fuzzy statistic 模糊统计

fuzzy structured element 模糊结构元

fuzzy-valued function 模糊值函数

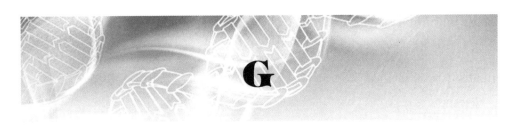

G

gain from medical treatment 医疗收益

gain on reversal of bad debts 坏账转回利益

game 博弈

game theory 博弈论

gastroenterology 肠胃病学

gastroscopy room 胃镜室

Gaussian distribution 高斯分布

general equilibrium 总体均衡

general health perceptions 总体健康感受

general hospital 总医院

general instruments 通用量表

general medical quality evaluation 总体医疗质量评价

general medicine 全科医学

General Office of the State Council 国务院办公厅

general physician 家庭(全科)医生

general practitioner 全科医师

general principle 总则

general standard 通用标准

generic drugs 通用药品

genetic epidemiology 遗传流行病学

genetics 遗传学

geographic factor 地理因素

geographic information system 地理信息系统

geographic jurisdiction 地域管辖权

geometric mean 几何均数

global budget 总额预算

global health budgets (GHB) 卫生总预算

Global Use of Strategies To open Occluded coronary arteries 全面应用多种策略以开放阻塞性冠状动脉

GMO food 转基因食品

goal-oriented evaluation 目标评价

gold standard 金标准

golden rule 黄金规则

good clinical practice (GCP) 药物临床试验管理规范

good in quality and low in price 质优价廉

good laboratory practice（GLP） 药物非临床研究质量管理

good manufacturing practice for drugs（GMP） 药品生产质量管理规范

goodness of fit 拟合优度

goodness of fit index 拟合优度指数

Gorton method 哥顿法

governing mechanism 治理机制

government bill 政府议案

government franchise 特许经营

government public relations 政府公共关系

government regulation 政府法规

government subsidy 政府补助

government supervision mode 政府督导模式

government welfare insurance scheme 公费医疗制度

graded nursing 分级护理

grant certification 授予证书

grant-in-aid fund 财政补贴基金

graph of frequency distribution 频数分布图

graph theory 图论

grass-roots supervision 基层监督

grey literature 灰色文献

grey relevancy degree 灰色关联度

gross domestic product 国内生产总值

gross premium 总保费

group decision support system（GDSS） 群体决策支持系统

group hospital 医院集团

group life insurance 团体人寿保险

group objective；collective objective 集体目标

group vision 团体愿景

grouping variable 分组变量

guarantee fund 保证金

gynecologist 妇科医师

gynecologist-in-charge 妇科主治医师

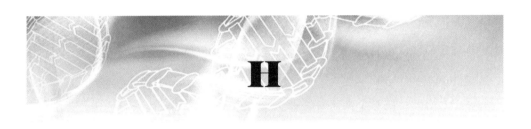

H

H test　H 检验

half cleanness section　半清洁区

Hall's three dimensional structure
霍尔三维结构

handbook of clinical evidence　临床
证据手册

handy service for the public　便民
服务

hardware construction　硬件建设

hardware resources　硬件资源

have both ability and political
integrity　德才兼备

Hawthorne experiment　霍桑实验

hazard function　风险函数

head nurse　护士长

health　健康

health account　卫生账户

health administrator training center
卫生管理人员培训中心

health and casualty insurance　健康
及意外险

health archive　健康档案

health authority　卫生行政部门

health bed resources　卫生床位资源

health behavior　健康行为

health benefits plan　健康福利计划

health bureau　卫生局

health care　保健

health care center　保健中心

health care consciousness　保健意识

health care cost　卫生服务成本

health care organization　保健组织

health care provider　医疗服务提
供方

health care quality improvement　医
疗质量改进法

health care reform　医疗改革

health care resources　卫生保健资源

health care system reform　卫生体
制改革

health consultation　卫生咨询

health consulting　健康咨询

health cost　健康价值

health economics　卫生经济学

health education　健康教育

health equipment resources　卫生设

备资源

health evaluation　卫生评价

health expenditure　卫生支出；卫生
费用

health expenditure per capita　人均
卫生费用

health field model　健康领域模型

health financing　卫生筹资

health fund resource　卫生经费资源

health global expenditure　卫生总
费用

health human resources　卫生人力
资源

health information network　健康信
息网络

health information system　卫生信
息系统

health insurance　健康保险

health insurance system　健康保险
制度

health investment　健康投资

health law　卫生法

health legislation　卫生立法

health lesion　健康损害

health maintenance organization
（HMO）　健康维持组织

health management　卫生管理

health measure　健康测量指标

health outcome　健康结果

health planning　卫生规划

health policy　卫生政策

health professional　卫生专业人员

health promotion　健康促进

health regulation　卫生法规

health resource　卫生资源

health resources distribution　卫生
资源配置

health risk factors appraisal
（HRFA）　健康危险因素评价

health risk index（HRI）　健康风险
指数

health sciences center　健康科学
中心

health service　卫生服务；卫生勤务

health service agency　卫生事业
机构

health service documents　卫勤文书

health service maneuvers　卫勤演习

health service reforms　卫生服务
改革

health service support　卫勤保障

health service system　卫生服务体系

health service training　卫勤训练

health states　健康状态

health station　保健站

health statistics　卫生统计学

health status　健康状况

health supervision　卫生监督

health surveillance　健康监视

health system　卫生系统

health technology　卫生技术

health technology assessment　卫生
技术评估

health technology man-power in
preliminary level　基层卫生技术
人才

health utility index　健康效用指数

healthcare administration　医疗卫生
行政管理

Healthcare Associations　医疗保健
协会

healthcare delivery system　医疗服
务提供体系

Healthcare Information and
Management Systems Society
（HIMSS）　医疗信息与管理系统
协会

health-related quality of life
（HRQL）　健康相关生命质量

heart function examination room
心功能室

Helicobacter pylori（Hp）　幽门螺
杆菌

hemodialysis machine　血液透析机

hemodialysis room　血透室

hemodialysis（HD）　血液透析

herd immunity　群体免疫力

heterogeneous product　异质产品

hierarchical clustering analysis　系
统聚类

hierarchical data model　层次数据
模型

hierarchical management　分级管理

hierarchical management and
accreditation of hospital　医院分
级管理和评审

hierarchical model　层次模型

high altitude sickness　高原病

high court of justice　高级法院

high input；high consuming　高投
入、高消耗

high level　高层次

high quality capital　优质资产

high quality service　优质服务

high-tech industry　高技术产业

histogram　直方图

historical controlled trial　历史性对
照研究

holding for treatment　留治

holding-room for severely wounded　危重伤员观察室

holistic care quality evaluation　整体护理质量评价

holistic effect　整体效应

home health care　居家护理

home medical service　家庭医疗服务

homogeneity of variance　方差齐性

homogeneity of variance test　方差齐性检验

horizontal equity　横向公平

horizontal integration　水平整合

horizontal relation　横向联系

horizontal transmission　横向传播；水平传播

hospital　医院

hospital accounting system　医院会计制度

hospital administrative department　医院管理部门

hospital administrative management　医院行政管理

hospital architecture　医院建筑

hospital asset　医院资产

hospital auditing　医院审计

hospital behavior culture　医院行为文化

hospital benefits　医院福利费

hospital building combination　医院建筑组合形式

hospital building equipment system　医院建筑设备系统

hospital building management　医院建筑管理

hospital capital　医院资本

hospital capital management　医院资本运营

hospital capital recomposition　医院资产重组

hospital characteristics　医院特性

hospital communication system　医院通信系统

hospital comprehensive benefits evaluation　医院综合效益评价

hospital computerized information system　医院计算机信息系统

hospital cost control　医院成本控制

hospital cost management　医院成本管理

hospital creditor's rights　医院债权

hospital cultural community　医院文化共同体

hospital culture   医院文化

hospital culture conception   医院文化观念

hospital culture network   医院文化网络

hospital culture of safety   医院安全文化

hospital culture scale   医院文化规模

hospital culture shock   医院文化冲突

hospital design and construction   医院设计和建设

hospital development   医院发展

hospital development strategy   医院发展战略

hospital drainage system   医院排水制度

hospital economics accounting   医院经济核算

hospital economics management   医院经济管理

hospital environment   医院环境

hospital environment and hygiene management   医院环境与卫生学管理

hospital equipment   医院设备

hospital equipment classification   医院设备分类

hospital evaluation standard   医院评价标准

hospital expansion   医院扩张

hospital expansion system   医院扩展系统

hospital expectation   医院期望

hospital external environment   医院外部环境

hospital external environment management   医院外环境管理

hospital facilities   医院设施

hospital fashion   医院风尚

hospital financial budgeting   医院财务预算

hospital firefighting system   医院消防系统

hospital fixed assets   医院固定资产

hospital for prisoners of war   战俘医院

hospital functional block   医院功能分区

hospital functional structure   医院职能机构

hospital fund management   医院基金管理

hospital human resources

management　医院人力资源管理

hospital hygienic management　医院
卫生学管理

hospital infection　医院感染

hospital infection control　医院感染
控制

hospital infection management　医
院感染管理

hospital infection monitoring　医院
感染监测

hospital infection rate　院内感染率

hospital information　医院信息

hospital information management
医院信息管理

hospital information system　医院信
息系统

hospital internal environment　医院
内部环境

hospital internal environment
management　医院内环境管理

hospital leadership　医院领导

hospital leadership system　医院领
导体制

hospital library　医院图书馆

hospital logistic management　医院
后勤管理

hospital logistics assurance　医院后

勤保障

hospital logistics management system
医院后勤管理体制

hospital macroscopic control and
adjustment　医院宏观调控

hospital management　医院管理

Hospital Management Association
医院管理学会

hospital management information
system　医院管理信息系统

hospital management standard　医
院管理标准

hospital management standardization
医院标准化管理

hospital management strategy　医院
经营管理战略

hospital management structure　医
院管理架构

hospital management system　医院
管理系统

hospital material management　医院
物资管理

hospital material quota management
医院物资定额管理

hospital matter culture　医院物质
文化

hospital morals　医院道德

hospital nature culture 医院本质
文化

hospital noise 医院噪声

hospital nursing management 医院
护理管理

hospital operation cooperation 医
院经营合作

hospital operation management 医
院经营管理

hospital operation system 医院运行
系统

hospital operational decision 医院
经营决策

hospital output index 医院产出指标

hospital performance assessment
system 医院绩效评估体系

hospital performance management
医院绩效管理

hospital performance management
evaluation 医院绩效管理评价

hospital performance management
system 医院绩效管理体系

hospital performance measurement
tools 医院绩效测量工具

hospital personnel organization 医
院人员编制

hospital philosophy 医院哲学

hospital price index 医院价格指数

hospital proprietary right 医院所
有权

hospital quality 医院质量

hospital quality control 医院质量
管理

hospital quality management systems
医院质量管理体系

hospital quality satisfaction 医院质
量满意度

hospital quality standardization 医
院质量标准化

hospital scale 医院规模

hospital sewage 医院污水

hospital spiritual culture 医院精神
文化

hospital standard 医院标准

hospital standard system 医院标准
体系

hospital statistical index 医院统计
指标

hospital statistics 医院统计

hospital strategy 医院战略

hospital strategy management 医院
战略管理

hospital strategy priority 医院战略
重点

hospital stratified management 医院分级管理

hospital structure 医院结构

hospital supply and distribution system 医院供应和分配系统

hospital support system 医院支持系统

hospital system engineering 医院系统工程

hospital technical management 医院技术管理

hospital tenet 医院宗旨

hospital traffic system 医院交通运输系统

hospital war preparation 医院战备

hospital waste-water disposal 医院污水处理

hospitalization 住院

hospitalization insurance policy 医疗保险政策

hospitalization insurance policy analysis 医疗保险政策分析

household;family 家庭

housing allowance 住房津贴

housing distribution 住房分配

housing reform 住房改革

housing subsidies 住房补贴

human capital 人力资本

human capital approach 人力资本法

human development index 人类发展指数

human relation 人际关系

human resource management 人力资源管理

human resource management of logistics department 后勤人事管理

human resource planning 人力资源规划

human resources 人力资源

human rights 人权

human-computer interaction 人-机对话

humanistic service 人性化服务

human-oriented 以人为本

human-oriented hospital culture 医院人本文化

hygienic standard;sanitary standard 卫生标准

hygieology;hygiology 卫生学

hyperbaric oxygen therapy center 高压氧舱治疗中心

hypothesis 假设

hypothesis test　假设检验

hypothetical scenarios　假设情境

hysteresis；retard　迟滞

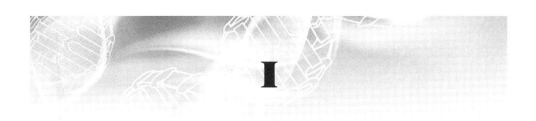

I

iatrogenic diseases 医源性疾病

International Classification of
Diseases 10（ICD-10） 国际疾病分
类标准编码 10

ideal weight 理想体重

identification 界定

identification of customer
requirements 顾客要求的识别

idle assets 闲置资产

illegal and unjustifiable funds and
charges 不合法、不合理资金筹集
和收费

immanent contradiction 内在矛盾

immaterial assets；nonphysical assets
无形资产

immunity 豁免权

impartiality；equity 公正性

impatient services 住院服务

implement phase 实施阶段

implementation 实施

implementation procedure 实施
程序

implicit cost 隐性成本

import license system 进口许可证
制度

improvement 改进；好转

in good faith 诚信

incidence density 发病密度

incidence of disease 发病率

incidence of infection 感染发病率

incidence of malpractice 医疗事故
发生率

incidence rate 发病率

incinerator 焚烧炉

income 收入

income elasticity 收入弹性

income elasticity of demand 需求
收入弹性

income from medical services 医疗
收入

income from property 产权收益

income per capita 人均收入

income tax expense 所得税费用

incoming fee per outpatient and
emergency patient 门急诊人均
费用

incomplete cost　不完全成本

incorporation intelligence　团队智商

increasing return to scale　报酬递增规律

increasing returns to scale　规模报酬递增

increment asset　增量资产

increment capital　增量资本

incremental analysis　增量分析

incremental cost effectiveness ratio　增量成本效果比

incubation　潜伏

incubation period　潜伏期

indemnity　补偿费

independent accounting　独立核算

independent operation　自主运营

independent variable　自变量

index of average wage　平均工资指数

index of outpatient quality　门诊质量指标

index on medical treatment quality　医疗质量评价指标

indications for evacuation　后送适应证

indictment　起诉

indifference curve　无差异曲线

indifferent　无差别

indirect application of international standard　国际标准的间接应用

indirect approach　间接法

indirect benefit　间接效益

indirect burden　间接经济负担

indirect causal association　间接因果联系

indirect cost　间接成本

indirect financing instrument　间接融资手段

indirect labor　间接人工

indirect nursing　间接护理

individual clinical expertise　个人临床专长

individual cultivation　个人修炼

individual demand curve　个人需求曲线

individual demand function　个人需求函数

individual development plan（IDP）个人发展计划

individual income tax　个人所得税

individual medical insurance account　个人医疗账户

individual opinion　个人见解

individual vision　个人愿景

individual wisdom   个人智慧

individualism   个人主义

individualization   个体化

induced abortion room   人工流产室

induced demand   诱导需求

induction   归纳法

industrial data processing   综合数据
处理系统

industrial economics   工业经济

industrial layout；industrial
distribution   产业布局

industrialization of hospital logistics
service   医院后勤服务产业化

industries and enterprises in dire
straits   特困行业和企业

industry   产业；行业

industry structure   产业结构

inefficiency   缺乏效率

inelastic   缺乏弹性的

infant mortality rate   婴儿病死率

infant mortality rate in hospital   院
内新生婴儿病死率

infection control   感染控制

infection control committee   感染控
制委员会

infection source   传染源

infectious disease report system   疫
情报告系统

infectious disease reporting   传染病
报告

infectious disease surveillance   传染
病监测

infectious disease；contagious
diseases   传染病

infinite population   无限总体

inflation   通货膨胀

inflection point   拐点

influence each other   相互影响

informal planning   非正式计划

informal system   非正式系统

informant   知情人

information   信息

information access   信息访问

information accounting   情报会计

information acquisition   信息获取

information asymmetry   信息非对
称性

information bias   信息偏倚

information carrier   信息载体

information collection   信息收集

information conversion   信息转换

information cost   信息成本

information distribution   信息分布

information economics   信息经济

information encoding　信息编码

information feedback　信息反馈

information flow　信息流

information handling　信息处理

information management　信息管理

information method　信息方法

information organization　信息组织

information output　信息输出

information planning　信息规划

information policy and law　信息政策与法规

information processing　信息加工

information processing system　信息处理系统

information quantity　信息量

information receiver　信息接收者

information resources management　信息资源管理

information retrieval　信息检索

information revolution　信息革命

information science　信息科学

information service　信息服务

information share　知识共享

information society　信息化社会

information source　信息资源

information storage　信息储存

information system　信息系统

information system architecture　信息体系结构

information technology　信息技术

information theory　信息论

information transmission　信息传递

informatization management　信息化管理

informed consent　知情同意

infrastructure　基础设施

inheritance　遗传

initial condition　初始条件

initiation　启动

injection room　注射室

innovation　创新

inpatient　住院患者

inpatient declaration　住院申报

in-patient department　住院部

input　输入

input-output　投入-产出

input-output model　投入-产出模型

inspection and control of quality　质量检控

inspection body　检验机构

inspection of quality conformity　质量一致性检验

inspection record　检验记录

Institute of Military Medicine　军事

医学研究所

institution；system　制度

institutional arrangement　制度安排

institutional design　制度设计

institutional economics　制度经济学

institutional guarantee　制度性保障

instrument　仪器

instrument room　仪器室

instrumental leader　指导型领导

insurable interest　保险利益

insurance　保险

insurance agent　保险代理人

insurance broker　保险经纪人

insurance claim　保险理赔

insurance company　保险公司

insurance coverage　保险范围

insurance evaluation　保险评估

insurance for the unemployed　失业保险

insurance fund　保险基金

insurance industry　保险业

insurance liability　保险责任

insurance market　保险市场

insurance mechanism　保险机制

insurance obligation　保险义务

insurance relations　保险关系

insurance statistics　保险统计

insurance storage　保险储备

insured　被保险方

insurer　保险方

intangible benefit　隐性效益

intangible capital　无形资本

integrated delivery system（IDS）　整体服务系统

integrated nursing　整体护理

integration　整合

integration medicine with authority　医政合一

integrity　完整性

intellectual property right（IPR）　知识产权

intelligence　智力；智能

intelligent assets　智力资产

intelligent decision support system（IDSS）　智能决策支持系统

intelligentization　智能化

intensive care unit　重症监护室

intensive development model　集约型模式

intensive management of hospital logistics service　医院后勤服务集约化

intensive micro-management　微观核算型管理

interaction　交互作用

interest rate　利息率

interest revenue　利息收入

inter-laboratory test comparisons
　实验室间的试验比较

intermediate goods　中间产品

intern　实习医师

internal activity　内部活动

internal audit　内部审核；内部审计

internal communication　内部沟通

internal dose　内剂量

internal environment　内部环境

internal evaluation　内部评价

internal factor　内部因素

internal governing structure　内部治
　理结构

internal hospital audit　医院内部
　审计

internal motive　内在动力

internal quality audits　内部质量
　审核

internal rate of return　内部收益率

internal validity　内在真实性

internally controlled standard　内控
　标准

international cooperation　国际合作

International Society for Quality in

Health Care（ISQHC）　国际医疗
质量协会

International Society of
　Pharmacoeconomics and Outcomes
　Research　国际药物经济学与结果
　研究协会

International Standard　国际标准

International Standardization
　Organization（ISO）　国际标准化
　组织

internship　实习

inter-organizational relations　组织
　间关系

interpersonal skills　人际交往能力

inter-rater reliability　测量评估者间
　信度

interval estimation　区间估计

intervention　干预

interventional procedures　干预措施

interviewer bias　调查者偏倚

intraclass correlation coefficient
　（ICC）　组内相关系数

intractable case　疑难病例

intra-rater reliability　测量评估者内
　信度

introspective method　内省法

invalid intervention　无效干预

invasive manipulation   侵入性操作

invention   发明

inventories   存货

inventory   存量;库存

inventory turnover/turns   库存(资
金)周转次数

inverse matrix   逆矩阵

investigation analysis   调查分析

investigation;investigate;inquire
into   调查

investment   投资

investment company   投资公司

investment income   投资收益

investment loss   投资损失

invisible cost   无形成本

irregular education   非正规教育

irresistible factors   不可抗拒的因素

ISO 9001 standard   ISO 9001 标准

ISO standard   ISO 标准

isocost line   等成本线

isolate;isolation   隔离

isolation and disinfection   隔离消毒

isolation ward   隔离病房

isoprofit curve   等利润曲线

isoquant curve   等产量曲线

item   项目

item-based cost accounting   医疗项
目成本核算

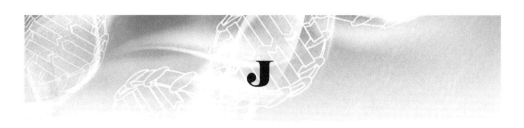

J

Japanese Standards Association 日本标准协会

job analysis 岗位分析

job burnout 工作倦怠

job design 工作设计

job training of personnel 人员岗位培训

Joint Commission on Accreditation of Healthcare Organization 卫生服务机构资格认证联合委员会

Joint Technical Committee 联合技术委员会

joint-stock hospital 股份制医院

joint-stock system 股份制

journal of statistical source 统计源期刊

judgement 判定

judgmental sampling 判断抽样

judicial act 司法法案

judicial documents 司法文书

judicial interpretation 司法解释

judicial organizations 司法机关

jurisprudence 法学

jurist 法学家

K

key discipline　重点学科

key role；core role　核心角色

killed in action　阵亡

kinds of medical care　救治种类

knowledge acquisition　知识获取

knowledge denseness　知识密集

knowledge economy　知识经济

knowledge flow sheet　知识流程

knowledge management　知识管理

knowledge renewal　知识更新

knowledge structure　知识结构

knowledge transmission　知识传递

Kruskal-Wallis H test　克鲁斯卡尔-
沃利斯 H 检验

kurtosis　峰度

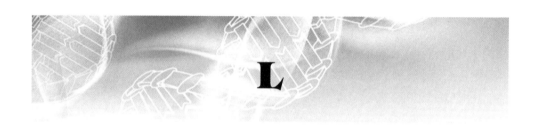

L

labor and social security 劳动和社会保障

labor cost 劳务费

labor force 劳动力

labor health service 劳保医疗

labor insurance scheme 劳保医疗制度

laboratory 实验室

laboratory assessment 实验室评定

laboratory assessor 实验室评定者

laboratory certification 实验室认证

laboratory information system 实验室信息系统

laboratory of immunology 免疫实验室

laboratory qualification 实验室鉴定

laboratory technician 实验员

labour insurance 劳动保险费

labour room 待产室

laid-off workers 下岗职工

laissez faire 自由放任

land 土地

language bias 语言偏倚

large scale medical institution 大型医疗单位

latent infection 隐性感染

latin squares design 拉丁方设计

lavation equipment 洗涤设备

law committee 法律委员会

law enforcement 法律的实施

law of demand 需求定理

law of demand and supply 供需法

law of diminishing marginal rate of substitution 边际替代递减法则

law of diminishing marginal return 边际收益递减规律

law of diminishing marginal utility 边际效用递减法则

law of downward-sloping demand 需求向下倾斜规律

law of increasing cost 成本递增法则

law of large number 大数法则

law of one price 单一价格法则

law of scarcity 稀缺法则

law report 判例汇编

law supervision　法律监督

law；legal　法律

law-based management　依法管理

lawyer notarization　律师公证

leader　领导者

leader behavior　领导行为

leadership role　领导角色

Leading Group of Birth Control　计划生育领导小组

learning hospital　学习型医院

learning organization　学习型组织

learning society　学习型社会

learning system　学习制度

least sum of squares　最小二乘

lecturer　讲师

legal　合法的

legal interests　合法权益

legal norms　法律规范

legal obligation　法律责任

legality；legitimacy　合法性

legislation　立法

legislative interpretation　立法解释

legislator　立法者

legitimatize　合法化

liability；obligation　义务

license　许可证

license for pharmaceutical trading　药品经营许可证

licensed pharmacist　执业药师

life cycle　生命周期

life cycle cost　寿命周期费用

life expectancy　期望寿命

life expectancy free of disability　无残疾期望寿命

life insurance　人寿保险

life quality index　生活质量指数

life subsidy　生活补助

life table　寿命表

life years　生存年数

lifelong learning　终身学习

lifestyle　生活方式

lifetime pursuit　终生追求

likelihood ratio　似然比

likelihood ratio test　似然比检验

limitation of payments　赔偿限额

limited budget　预算约束

line graph　线图

linear　直线的；线性的

linear correlation　直线相关

linear demand function　线性需求函数

linear forecasting　直线趋势预测

linear programming　线性规划

linear programming mathematical

model   线性规划数学模型

linear regression   直线回归

liquidity   流动性

literature retrieval   文献检索

litigation   诉讼

live and work in peace and
    contentment   安居乐业

location of injury   伤部

logic   逻辑

logical control   逻辑控制

logistic office   总务科

Logistic regression   逻辑斯谛回归

Logistic regression model   逻辑斯谛
    回归模型

logistics   后勤

logistics department   后勤保障部门

logistics equipment management   后
    勤设备管理

logistics management   后勤管理

logistics material management   后勤
    物资管理

logistics material supply   后勤物资供应

logistics service company   后勤服务
    公司

longitudinal survey   纵向调查

long-term average cost   长期平均
    成本

long-term bond investments   长期债
    券投资

long-term disability   长期失能

long-term equilibrium   长期均衡

long-term equity investments   长期
    股权投资

long-term forecasting   长期预测

long-term investments   长期投资

long-term liabilities   长期负债

long-term loans payable   长期借款

long-term marginal cost   长期边际
    成本

long-term orientation   长期导向

long-term planning   长期规划

long-term prepaid rent   长期预付
    租金

long-term real estate in-vestments
    长期不动产投资

long-term total cost   长期总成本

look up; consult   查阅

loss of state assets   国有资产流失

loss ratio   赔付率

loss to follow-up bias   失访偏倚

loss to follow-up; loss to observation
    失访

low-cost consuming products   低值
    易耗品

M

machanism 机制

macro-control 宏观调控

macro-control targets 宏观调控目标

macro-decision 宏观决策

macro distribution 宏观配置

macroeconomic 宏观经济

macroeconomic model 宏观经济模型

macroeconomic targets 宏观经济目标

macro-management 宏观管理

main effect 主效应

maintain 维修

maintain value 保值

maintenance 维护

malnutrition 营养不良

managed care 管理式医疗;管理型保健

management accounting 管理会计

management by exception 例外管理法

management by objectives 目标管理

management function 管理职能

management information system 管理信息系统

management model 管理模式

management of antisepsis 消毒管理

management of epidemic situation 疫情管理

management of operation room 手术室管理

management of organization 组织管理

management of outpatient department 门诊管理

management position 管理地位

Management Regulations on Sanitation Regulation at Public Places 公共场所卫生管理条例

management representative 管理者代表

management responsibility 管理职责

management review 管理评审

management review control
　　procedure　管理评审控制程序

management structure　经营结构

management system　管理体系

management value concept　管理价
　　值观

manager　经理

managerial benefit　管理效益

managerial decision　管理决策

managerial environment　管理环境

managerial grid　管理方格图

managerial perspective　管理视野

managing path　管理流程

man-hour　工时

manpower allocation　人力配置

manpower input　人力投入

marginal analysis　边际分析

marginal benefit　边际收益

marginal benefit product　边际收益
　　产品

marginal cost　边际成本

marginal cost of factor　边际要素
　　成本

marginal returns　边际回报

marginal revenue　边际收益

marginal salaries　边际薪酬

marginal social benefit　社会边际

收益

marginal social cost　社会边际成本

marginal utility　边际效用

margins；collateral　保证金；附属担
　　保金

mark of conformity　合格标志

mark of conformity certification
　　合格认证标志

mark of safety certification　安全认
　　证标志

marker of triage　分类标志

market behavior　市场行为

market competition　市场竞争

market concentration ratio　市场集
　　中率

market-driving type　市场趋动型

market economy　市场经济

market factor　市场要素

market failure　市场失灵

market mechanism　市场机制

market of medical service　医疗服
　　务市场

market power　市场力

market regulation　市场法规

market research　市场调查

market scale　市场规模

market segmentation　市场细分

market share   市场占有率

market structure   市场结构

marketing   市场营销

marketing policy   市场政策

marketing strategy   营销策略

Markov model   马尔可夫模型

marriage   婚姻

marriage boom   结婚高峰

match   匹配

matched case control study   配对病例对照研究

matched t-test   配对 t 检验

matching   配对

matching environment   环境匹配

material amenities   生活待遇

material balanced table   物资平衡表

material capital   实物资本

material classification   物资分类

material needs   物质的需要

material procurement   物资的采购

material requirement   物资需要量

material resources   物力

material stocks   库存物资

material storage   物资储备量

material storehouse   物资库

maternal and child health（MCH）妇幼保健

maternal and infant care（MIC）母婴保健

maternal mortality rate   孕产妇病死率

maternity ward   产科病房

mathematical model   数学模型

mathematical model of decision   决策数学模型

maximal aggregate loss   最大损失总额

maximal loss principle   最大损失原理

maximization   极大化

maximum liability limit   最高责任限额

maximum likelihood   最大似然法

mean   平均数

mean operation time   平均手术时间

mean square   均方

mean value principle   均值原理

measure   测量

measure of quantity   量化测量

measure of time   时间测量

measurement control system   测量控制体系

measurement data   计量资料

measurement error   测量误差

measurement of hospital culture　医院文化评测

measurement of work time　工时测定法

measurement variation　测量变异

measuring bias　测量偏倚

mechanism adjustment　机制调整

mechanism of hospital culture　医院文化机制

mechanism of pharmaceutical market　医药市场机制

mechanism of procurement　采购机制

median　中位数

median survival time　中位生存时间

medicaid program　医疗补助计划

medical nursing center　医疗护理中心

medical accident appraisal　医疗事故鉴定

medical activities　医疗活动

medical administration　医疗管理

medical administration division　医务部(处)

medical and teaching administration　医教部

medical battalion　卫生营

medical brigade　卫生旅

medical care quality　医护质量

medical care system　医疗制度

medical center　医疗中心

medical company　卫生连

medical cooperation system　医疗合作制度

medical corpsman　连卫生员

medical cosmetic center　医学美容中心

medical cost　医疗成本

medical cost accounting　医疗成本核算

medical cost control　医疗成本控制

medical cost management　医疗成本管理

medical decision making　医疗决策

medical demand　医疗需求

Medical Department of General Logistics Department of CPLA　总后勤部卫生部

medical detachment　医疗队

medical devices　医疗器械

medical dispute　医疗纠纷

medical division　卫生处

medical document　医疗文书

medical economic policy　卫生经济

政策

medical education and training　医疗教育和培训

medical effect　医疗效果

medical equipments　医疗设备

medical error　医疗差错

medical ethics　医学伦理学

medical evacuation　医疗后送

medical evacuation system　医疗后送体制

medical evaluation　医疗评价

medical expenditure　医疗费用

medical expense　医疗费

medical health care　医疗保健

medical image center　医学影像中心

medical informatics　医学信息学

medical information　医学情报

medical institutions　医疗机构

medical instrument repairing shop　医疗器械检修所

medical insurance　医疗保险

medical insurance institution　医疗保险机构

medical insurance law　医疗保险法

medical insurance management　医疗保险管理

medical Insurance management information system（MIMIS）　医疗保险管理信息系统

medical insurance overage card　医疗保险卡

medical insurance premium　医疗保险费

medical insurance reform in urban altd　城镇职工医疗保险制度改革

medical insurance science　医疗保险学

medical insurance system　医疗保险制度

medical linear accelerator　医用直线加速器

medical loss ratio　医疗损失比例

medical malpractice　医疗事故

medical market analysis　医疗市场分析

medical market environment　医疗市场环境

medical materials　卫生材料

medical model　医学模式

medical obligation　医疗责任

medical order　医疗秩序

medical personnel；medical staff　医务人员

medical post　卫生所

medical practice　医疗实践

medical professionals　医学技术人员

medical psychology　医学心理学

medical quality　医疗质量

medical quality control　医疗质量控制

medical quality evaluation system　医疗质量评价体系

medical quality management　医疗质量管理

medical quality standard　医疗质量标准

medical record　病历;病案

medical reference range　医学参考值范围

medical resource　医疗资源

medical resource allocation　医疗资源配置

medical resource structure　医疗资源结构

medical right infringement lawsuit　医疗侵权诉讼

medical risk　医疗风险

medical risk management　医疗风险管理

medical safety　医疗安全

medical safety management　医疗安全管理

medical safety precaution　医疗安全防范

medical science and technology　医学科学技术

medical science and technology progress　医学科技进步

medical section　卫生科

medical service market　医疗服务市场

medical service quality　医疗服务质量

medical service unit　卫勤分队

medical services group　医疗集团

medical sociology　医学社会学

medical statistics　医学统计学

medical supplies for first aid in war　战救药材

medical supply　药材供应

medical supply accounting　药材核算

medical supply standard　药材供应标准

medical supply statistics　药材统计

medical support group　医疗保障组

medical system　医疗体系

medical tag　伤票

medical technique standard　医疗技术标准

medical technology　医学技术

medical technology resources　医学技术资源

Medical Treatment Administrative Division　医疗管理局

medical ward　内科病房

medical waste　医疗废物

Medicare　美国老年人医疗保险计划

Medicare Prescription Drug Benefit　美国老年人医疗保险处方药补偿计划

medicare system reform　医疗制度改革

medication treatment　药物治疗

medicinal chemistry　药物化学

medicine　医学

Medicine and Supplies Division　药品器材局

medicine intellectual property rights　医药知识产权

medico technical method standard　医疗技术方法标准

medico technical operation standard　医疗技术操作标准

medico technical standard system　医疗技术标准体系

medifund　保健基金

medisave　保健储蓄

medishield　健保双全

medium scale　中等规模

medium value　平均值

member of certification system　认证体系的成员

mental activism　心理能动性

mental activity　心理活动

mental handicap　精神障碍

mental health　心理健康

mental hospital　精神病院

mental impairment　精神损害

mental mode　心智模式

mental phenomenon　心理现象

mental process　心理过程

mental state　精神状态

merger　兼并

merger and reorganization　兼并重组

meta analysis　荟萃分析

metrological characteristic　计量特性

metrological confirmation　计量确认

microbe　微生物

micro-control 微观调控

micro-decision 微观决策

mid-term forecasting 中期预测

mid-term planning 中期规划

midwife 接生员

migrant worker 外来工

migrant workers in cities 进城务工
农民

military establishments 军事机构

military health service administration
军队卫生事业管理

military hospital 军队医院

military medical college 军事医
学院

military medical supply
administration 军队药材管理

military medical university 军医
大学

military medicine 军事医学

minimum balance 最小库存余量

minimum cost analysis 最低成本
分析

minimum wage 最低工资

minimum wage system 最低工资
制度

minister；superintendent 部长

Ministry of Finance 财政部

Ministry of Labour and Social
Security 劳动和社会保障部

Ministry of Public Health 卫生部

misallocation of resources 资源误置

misclassification bias 归类偏倚

missing 失踪

missing report 漏报

mission 使命

mixed cost 混合成本

mixed economy 混合经济

mixed mode 复合型

mobile reserve of medical supplies
药材流动储备

mobilization of health service
resources 卫勤机动力量

model parameter 模型参数

model selection 模式选择

moderate scale 适度规模

modern hospital 现代医院

modern human resources
management 现代人力资源管理

modern medical model 现代医学
模式

modern nursing management 现代
医院护理管理

modern operational management
现代经营管理

modernization of hospital logistics
医院后勤现代化

monitoring 监测;监控

monopolistic competition 垄断性
竞争

monopolized industry 垄断行业

monopoly 垄断

monopoly price 垄断价格

monopoly profit 垄断利润

monopsony 买方垄断

Monte Carlo simulation 蒙特卡洛
模拟

monthly report of medical statistics
卫生统计月报

moral construction in the hospital
culture 医院文化的道德建设

moral hazard 道德损害

moral norms 道德规范

morbidity 发病率

mortality 病死率

mother-infant rooming-in 母婴同室

motivation 激励

motivation measures 激励措施

motivation mechanism 激励机制

motivator 激励因素

motive 动机

movement of population 人口流动

multi-element system 多要素系统

multifactorial disease 多因子病

multilateral arrangement 多边协议

multi-level system 多层次系统

multi-objective decision 多目标决策

multiple comparison 多重比较

multiple correlation coefficient 复
相关系数

multiple linear regression 多元线性
回归

multiple publication bias 多重发表
偏倚

multiple sampling 多次抽样

multistage sampling 多级抽样

multivariate regression forecasting
method 多元性回归预测法

multiway 多向

mutation theory 突变论

mutual control 相互制约

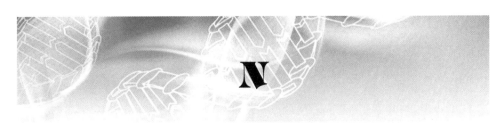

narrative method　叙述法

Nash equilibrium　纳什均衡

national asset transformation　国有资产转化

national body　国家团体

national compulsory insurance　国民义务保险

national culture　民族文化

national drugs policies system　国家药品政策体系

national health service（NHS）　国家卫生服务

National Institute for Clinical Excellence（NICE）　国家临床标准研究所

national treatment　国民待遇

natural growth rate　自然增长率

natural law　自然规律

natural losses　自然损耗

natural monopoly　自然垄断

natural resource　自然资源

natural system　自然系统

navy hospital　海军医院

NBC defense group　三防小组

necessary condition　必要条件

necessities　必需品

need　需要

need analysis　需要评估

need assessment　需求评估

needs for self-actualization　自我实现的需要

negative binomial distribution　负二项式分布

negative feedback　负反馈

negative population growth（NPG）　人口负增长

negative predictive value　阴性预测值

negligence；delinquency　过失

negotiation　协商

neonate　新生儿

neonate intensive care unit　新生儿重症监护室

net asset　净资产

net benefit（NB）　净效益

net demand　净需求

net income or loss for current period
本期损益

net premium   纯保险费

net premium principle   净保费原理

net present value   净现值

net revenue per physician   每个医师
的净收益

network chart and network planning
网络图与网络计划

network management system   网络
系统管理

network structure   网络结构

neurologist   神经科专家

new and special drugstore   新特
药房

new drug application   新药申请

new drug approval   新药审批

new field of technical activity   技术
活动新领域

new idea   新观念

newly rising industry   新兴产业

news media   新闻媒介

noise-induced deafness   噪声引起
耳聋

non-performing loans   不良贷款

non-battle casualties   非战斗减员

non-battle injury   非战斗外伤

noncompetitive   非竞争性

non-governmental organization
（NGO）   非政府组织

non-infectious diseases   非传染性
疾病

nonlinear pricing   非线性定价

nonlinear regression forecasting
method   非线性回归预测法

non-operating revenue   营业外收入

non-periodic inspection   不定期检查

non-procedural decision   非程序化
决策

non-profit   非营利性

non-profit organization   非营利组织

non-profitable agency   非营利性
机构

non-randomized concurrent
controlled trial   非随机同期对照
试验

nonrecurring gain or loss   非经常营
业损益

non-response bias   无应答偏倚

non-routine decision   非常规型决策

non-state-owned legal person's shares
社会法人股

normal   正态

normal distribution   正态分布

normal goods　正常品

normal profit　正常利润

normality test　正态性检验

normative document　标准文件

normative economics　规范经济学

normative forecasting　规范性预测

nosocomial infection；hospital infection　医院内感染

Nottingham health profile　诺丁汉健康调查表

nuclear magnetic resonance（NMR）核磁共振

null hypothesis　无效假设

number of admission　入院人数

number of inpatients　住院人数

number of separation　出院患者数

number of visits　诊疗人次

number of wounded passed　伤员通过量

nurse　护士

nurse's duty room　护士值班室

nurse-in-charge　主管护师

nurse practitioner　护师

nursing　护理

nursing care activity　护理行为

nursing cost　护理成本

nursing department　护理部

nursing dispute　护理纠纷

nursing economics　护理经济学

nursing files　护理档案

nursing human resources　护理人力资源

nursing human resources allocation　护理人员配备

nursing human resources management　护理人力资源管理

nursing informatics　护理信息学

nursing management　护理管理

nursing management standard　护理管理标准

nursing management system　护理管理体制

nursing management technique　护理管理技巧

nursing manager　护理管理者

nursing mark　护理标识

nursing minimum data set　护理最小数据集

nursing model　护理模式

nursing procedure　护理程序

nursing processes　护理过程

nursing quality　护理质量

nursing quality appraisal　护理质量评估

nursing record   护理记录

nursing resources   护理资源

nursing risk   护理风险

nursing risk evaluation   护理风险
    评价

nursing risk event   护理风险事件

nursing risk handling   护理风险处理

nursing risk identification   护理风
    险识别

nursing safety   护理安全

nursing safety management   护理安
    全管理

nursing station   护士站

nursing task   护理任务

nutrition and food hygiene   营养与
    食品卫生学

nutritionist   营养师

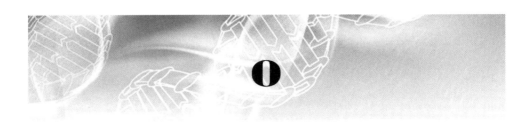

obedience　服从

object of insurance　保险标的物

objective evidence　客观证据

objective function　目标函数

objective risk　客观风险

objective world　客观世界

objects of financial management　财
　务管理对象

obligation of a patient　患者的义务

obligation to inform　告知义务

observation ward　观察室

observational bias　观察偏倚

observational studies　观察研究

observational study　观察性研究

obstetrician　产科医师

obstetrics and gynecology department
　妇产科

occupancy rate　占有率

occupancy rate of beds; sickbed
　average usage rate　平均病床利
　用率

occupancy rate of hospitals beds　病
　床使用率

occupational asthma　职业性哮喘

occupational cataract　职业性白内障

occupational disease　职业病

occupational fluorosis　工业性氟病

occupational psychology　职业心理

occupational therapist　作业治疗师
　（士）

oculist　眼科医师

odds　比数；比值

odds ratio　比值比

Office of Technology Assessment
　技术评估办公室

official compendium　行政纲领；法
　定纲要

oncologist　肿瘤科医师

on duty　出勤

one factor ANOVA　单因素方差
　分析

one sample/group t-test　单样本
　（组）t 检验

open procurement　公开采购

open tender　公开招标

open trial　开放试验

operating ability   经营才能

operating efficiency   运行效率;运营效率

operating revenue   营业收入

operation   手术

operation detachment   手术队

operation fee   手术费

operation management   经营管理

operation rate   手术率

operation research   运筹学

operation room   手术室

operation security   手术安全

operational costs   业务成本

operational mechanism   运行机制

operational model of service management   服务经营型管理

operational rear   战役后方

operational research   运筹学

operational style   运营方式

operational system   运营系统

ophthalmologist   眼科专家

ophthalmology   眼科学

opportunity   机会

opportunity cost   机会成本

optimal choice   最佳选择

optimal control   最优控制

optimal feasible   最优可行

optimal programme   最优方案

optimal resource allocation   最佳资源配置

optimal scale   最佳规模

optimization   优化

optimize allocation   优化配置

optimum allocation of medical resource   医疗资源优化配置

oral hospital   口腔医院

oral surgery   口腔外科

oral/dental sciences   口腔/牙科科学

order   有序

orderly competition   有序竞争

ordinary life insurance   普通人寿保险

organ transplantation   器官移植

organization   组织

organization image   组织形象

organization mission   组织任务

organization of financial management   财务管理组织

organization vision   组织愿景

organizational behavior   组织行为学

organizational culture   组织文化

organizational economics   组织经济学

organizational function　组织职能

organizational reform　组织变革

organizational strategy　组织战略

organizational structure　组织结构

original copy　资料原件

originality；creativity　创造力

orthogonal design　正交设计

orthopedist　矫形外科医师

osteopathic medicine　骨科医学

otology　耳科学

out of pocket　个人支付

outbreak　暴发；流行

outcome　转归

outcome evaluation　结果评价

outcomes　结果

outcomes nodes　结果节点

outcomes research　结果研究

out-patient　门诊患者

outpatient declaration　门诊申报

outpatient department of pediatrics　儿科门诊

outpatient injection room　门诊注射室

outpatient nurse's office　门诊护士办公室

outpatient office　门诊办公室

outpatient service　门诊

outpatient services　门诊服务

outpatient visits　门诊人次数

output　输出

output maximization　产出最大化

outside the law　超出法律范围

over effect　过度作用

overall budget　总预算

overall competitiveness　综合竞争力

overall medical fund in all society　社会统筹医疗基金

overall perspective；overall views　大局观念

overall planning　统筹规划

overall sales　总销售量

overall social joint relief　社会统筹

overdraft　透支

oversupply　过度供给

over-the-counter（OTC）　非处方药

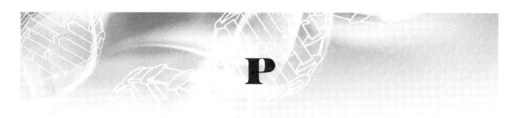

P

package of medical insurance 医疗保险范围

package treatment 袋装处理

paired comparison 平行比较法

panel 专门小组

paramedics 药剂人员

parameter 参数

parametric test 参数检验

Pareto criterion 帕累托标准

Pareto improvement 帕累托改进

Pareto optimality 帕累托优化

Pareto Principle 帕累托原理

partial cost 不完全成本

partial regression coefficient 偏回归系数

participative leadership 参与型领导

partner 工作伙伴

pass information 传递信息

passive immunity 人工被动免疫

passive management 被动管理

patent 专利

path analysis 路径分析

patient 患者

patient benefit 患者利益

patient-centred 以患者为中心

patient classification 患者分类

patient management 患者管理

patient preference 患者偏好

patient satisfaction 患者满意度

patient satisfaction appraisal 患者满意度评估

patient value perspective 患者价值观

patient's expected event rate 患者预期事件发生率

patient-reported outcomes（PRO）患者自报结果

patients the first 患者第一

pay as you go 现收现付

payment system 支付方式;偿付制度

payout 支出

payroll expense 薪资支出

Pearson correlation coefficient 皮尔逊相关系数

pediatrician 儿科医师

peer review   同行评价

peer review organization   同行审查组织

penalty；fine   罚款

pension   退休金；养老金

pension fund   退休基金

pensions to retired employees   离退休人员养老金

per capita   按人头支付

percent bar chart   百分比条图

percent sampling inspection   抽样检查百分比

percentage of unreported infectious diseases   传染病漏报率

percentile   百分位数

perfect positive correlation   完全正相关

performance   绩效

performance appraisal   绩效考核；绩效评估

performance evaluation   绩效评价

performance improvement（PI）   品质提升

performance management   绩效管理

performance measurement   业绩评价

performance review   绩效审查

perinatal   围生期

period of insurance   保险期限

periodic inspection   定期检验

periodical forecast   定时预测

perioperative period   围手术期

permanent population   常住人口

persisted learning   持续性学习

personal account   个人账户

personal income tax   个人所得税

personal injury   人身损害

personal insurance   人身保险

personal interest   个人利益

personal mastery   自我超越

personal responsibility   个人责任

personal savings insurance   个人储蓄保险

personal worth   个人价值

personalized service   个性化服务

personnel allocation   人员调配

personnel archives management   人事档案管理

personnel category   人员种类

personnel level   人员层次

personnel management   人事管理

personnel quality   人员素质

personnel quantity   人员数量

personnel structure 人员结构

personnel training 人员培训

persons at risk of exposure 高危人群

person-time analysis 人时分析

person-time of emergency visits 急诊人次数

perspective 角度

phannacoeconomics 药物经济学

pharmaceutical administration 药事管理

pharmaceutical administration committee 药事管理委员会

Pharmaceutical Benefits Scheme （PBS）药物保险计划

pharmaceutical bidding 药品招标

pharmaceutical care 药学保健

pharmaceutical education 药学教育

pharmaceutical management law 药品管理法

pharmaceutical marketing and management 药品营销与管理

pharmaceutical research and development 药品开发

pharmaceutical undertaking 药学事业

pharmacist 药师

pharmacist-in-charge 主管药师

pharmacoeconomics 药物经济学

pharmacoeconomics analysis 药物经济学分析

pharmacoepidemiology 药物流行病学

pharmacy 药房

pharmacy administration 药事管理学

pharmacy and therapeutics committee 药物和治疗委员会

pharmacy management 药房管理

pharmacy of hospital 医院药局

pharmacy practice 药学实践

pharmacy service 药学服务

pharmacy store 药库

phase Ⅰ clinical trial Ⅰ期临床试验

phased care 分级救治

philosophy of service 服务观念

phono-cardiography room 心音图室

physiatrist，rehabilitation physician 康复医师

physical and mental health 身心健康

physical check-up 健康检查

physical examination fee   检查费

physical form   实物形态

physical quality life index   生活质量指数

physical therapy   理疗

physician availability   医师的可获得性

physician practice management   医师行医管理

physiological monitoring system   生理监控系统

physiological needs   生理的需要

physiotherapist   理疗医师(士)

physiotherapy room   理疗室

picture archiving & communication system(PACS)   图像存储与通信系统

pie chart   饼图

pilot project   试点项目

pipeline transportation   管道运输

placebo   安慰剂

placebo effect   安慰剂效应

plan and manage as a whole   统筹管理

plan and prepare   筹划

plan of health service support   卫勤保障计划

plan，do，check，action cycle   PDCA 循环

planed immunity   计划免疫

planned economy   计划经济

planned results   预期结果

planning   规划

planning and financial division   计划财务处

planning management   计划管理

plaster room   石膏室

plastic surgeon   整形外科医师

platform   平台

point estimation   点估计

Poisson distribution   泊松分布

policy   保险单

policy analysis   政策分析

policy and code   政策法规

policy claim   政策主张

policy evaluation   政策评价

policy holder or proposer   投保人

policy impact analysis   政策影响分析

policy research   政策研究

polluted section   污染区

polyclinic   联合诊疗所

popularity；reputation   知名度

population   人口;群体;总体

population attributable risk 人群归因危险度

population attributable risk proportion 人群归因危险度比

population base 人口基数

population census 人口普查

population pyramid 人口年龄金字塔

population replacement level 人口更替水平

population statistics；demographics 人口统计

population studies 人口研究

population theory 人口理论

population-based cohort study 人群为基础的队列研究

position analysis 职位评价

positive feedback 正反馈

positive predictive value 阳性预测值

positive skewness distribution 正偏态分布

post alteration 岗位变动

post payment 后付制度

postal interview 信访

post marketing surveillance 上市后的监测

postoperative observation ward 术后观察室

post-surgery mortality 手术后死亡率

post-test odds 验后比

post-test probability 验后概率

potential 潜能

potential partner 潜在合作伙伴

potential years of life lost 潜在减寿年数

power 统计效能

power equipment 动力设备

power of a test 检验效能

power of attorney 委托权

power structure 权力结构

PR agencies 公关机构

practical demand 实际需要

practice of hospital culture 医院文化实践

practicing doctor；practicing physician 执业医师

practicing physicians law 执业医师法

precept value of cost（CPV） 成本贴现值

precision 精确性

prediction 预测

prediction of human resources   人力资源预测

pre-education and training for new staff members   新职工上岗前培训

preference   偏好

preferential policy   优惠政策

preferred provider organization（PPO）   优先者提供组织

pregnancy   妊娠

preliminary plan of health service support   卫勤保障预案

premarket control   市场前控制

premium   保险费

pre-natal care room   产前检查室

preoperative preparation room   术前准备室

prepaid expenses   预付费用

prepaid insurance   预付保险费

prepaid payroll   预付薪资

prepaid pension cost   预付退休金

prepaid rents   预付租金

preparation of normative document   标准文件的制订

prepayment   预付

prescription   处方

prescription drugs   处方药

present value   现值

preservation；storage   保管

pressure   压力

pre-test odds   验前比

pre-test probability   验前概率

prevalence   患病率

preventable risk   预防性风险

prevention   预防

prevention and control   预防和控制

prevention and health care network   预防保健网络

prevention and health care system   预防保健体制

prevention and supervision system   预防监督体制

prevention and treatment measures   防治措施

prevention of occupational diseases   职业病预防

prevention service   预防服务

preventive health service model   预防保健服务模式

preventive measures   预防措施

preventive medicine   预防医学

price   价格

price adjustment model   价格调整模型

price ceiling   最高限价

price consumption curve　价格消费曲线

price control　价格管制

price cut　削价

price difference　价格差别

price discrimination　价格歧视

price elasticity　价格弹性

price elasticity of demand　需求价格弹性

price elasticity of supply　供给价格弹性

price index　价格指数

price theory　价格理论

prices for medicines　药品定价

pricing　定价

pricing control of drugs　药品定价管制

pricing mechanism　价格机制

primary effect　首因效应

primary health and maternal & child health　基层卫生与妇幼保健

primary health care　初级卫生保健

primary health supervision　基层卫生监督

primary prevention　一级预防

primary preventive health care network　基层预防保健网络

primary research evidence　原始研究证据

primary sampling units　初级抽样单位

primary studies　原始研究

principal components analysis　主成分分析

principal-agent issues　委托-代理问题

private　民营

private benefit　个人效益

private capital　私人资本

private clinic　私人诊所

private cost　私人成本

private economy　私营经济

private goods　私人产品

private hospital　民营医院

private property　私人财产

privatization model　民营化模式

PR-minded　公关意识

probability　概率

probability of risk　危险率

probability sampling　概率抽样

procedure　程序

procedure law　诉讼法

process　过程

process control　过程控制

process evaluation　过程评价

process quality　环节质量

process utility　过程效用

procurement　采购

procurement of drugs　药品采购

procurement of medical supplies　药
材购买

procurement procedures　采购程序

producer equilibrium　生产者均衡

producer price;manufacturer price
出厂价

product　产品

product performance report　产品性
能报告

product security　产品安全

production capacity　生产能力

production domain　生产领域

production factors　生产要素

production function　生产函数

production oriented　生产导向

productive efficiency　生产效率

productivity　生产率

productivity of labor　劳动生产率

product-limited method　乘积极限法

professional ethics　职业道德

professor　教授

professor of pediatrics　儿科主任

医师

profit　利润

profit control　利润控制

profit distribution　利润分配

profit function　利润函数

profit maximization　利润最大化

profitability　利润率

profitable hospital　营利性医院

profits level　利润水平

prognosis　预后

prognostic factor　预后因素

prognostic index　预后指数

program evaluation research
technology　项目评估和研究技术

program manager　项目经理

programmed decision　程序决策

programming　程序化

progressive increase　递增

progressive reformation　渐进式
改革

promotion　促进作用;晋升

promotion assessment　晋升考核

property right　产权

property right connection　产权关系

proportion;ratio　比例

proportional mortality ratio（PMR）
比例死亡比

proportional or proportionate study
比例研究

proposal for health service support
卫勤保障建议

proposal of insurance   参保

proposed cost   建议成本

proprietary right   所有权

prospective payment system   预付
制度

prospective study   前瞻性研究

prospects   前景

protection against radiation   放射
防护

protection of medical supplies   药材
防护

protection; safe guard   防护

psychiatrist   精神病学专家

psychological dependence   精神依赖

psychological dimension   心理维度

psychological quality   心理素质

psychological stress   心理应激

psychology   心理学

psychomotor   心理运动

psychopath   精神变态者

psychophysical method   心理物理学
方法

psychophysics   心理物理学

psychosomatic relation   身心关系

psychotechnics   心理技术学

public administration model   公共管
理模式

public affairs   公共事务

public analysis   公众分析

public behavior   公众行为

public benefits   公共收益

public choice   公共选择

public choice theory   公共选择理论

public community psychology   公众
群体心理

public environment   公众环境

public finance   公共金融学

public goods   公共产品

public health   公共卫生

public health service   公费医疗

public health services   公共卫生
服务

public health undertaking   公共卫生
事业

public hospital   公立医院

public housing funding system   住房
公积金制度

public individual psychology   公众
个体心理

public opinion   公众舆论

public ownership　公有制

public policy　公共政策

public preference　公共偏好

public relation　公共关系

public relation consciousness　公共
关系意识

public relation goal　公共关系目标

public relations consulting　公共关
系咨询

public resources　公共资源

publication bias　发表偏倚

punish；sanction　制裁

purchase cost　购置费

purchase costs　订货成本

purchaser　购买者

purchasing power　购买力

Pygmalion effect　皮革马利翁效应

pyrogen reaction　热原反应

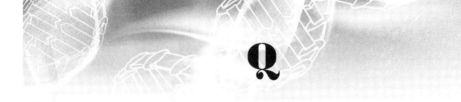

Q

qualification of personnel　人员资格

qualification process　鉴定过程

qualified product　合格品

qualitative analysis　定性分析

qualitative decision　定性决策

qualitative objective　定性目标

quality　质量

quality adjusted life year（QALY）
　质量调整生命年

quality arbitration　质量仲裁

quality assurance　质量保证

quality assurance system　质量保证
　体系

quality audit　质量审核

quality characteristic　质量特性

quality control　质量控制

quality control method　质量控制
　方法

quality control of specified diseases
　病种质量控制

quality control office　质控室

quality control system　质量控制
　体系

quality diagnosis　质量诊断

quality evaluation　质量评价

quality improvement　质量改进

quality index　质量指标

quality information control　质量信
　息控制

quality inspection　质量检验

quality management　质量管理

quality management system　质量管
　理体系

quality manual　质量手册

quality monitoring　质量监测；质量
　监督；质量监控

quality monitoring laboratory　质量
　检验室

quality objective　质量目标

quality of life　生命质量

quality of life benefit　生存质量效
　益法

quality of life index　生命质量指数

quality of products　产品质量

quality of service　服务质量

quality plan　质量计划

quality planning　质量策划

quality policy　质量方针

quality programs　质量纲领

quality records　质量记录

quality requirements　质量要求

quality standard　质量标准

quality supervision for approval　评价型质量监督

quality system　质量体系

quality system certification　质量体系认证

quantitative analysis　定量分析

quantitative data　定量资料

quantitative forecast　定量预测

quantitative objective　定量目标

quantitized assessment　量化评价

quantity of demand　需求量

quantity of life　生活数量

quantized appraisal　量化考核

quarantine　检疫

quarantine station　检疫所

quartile range　四分位数间距

quasi-randomized controlled trial　类随机对照试验

questionnaire　调查表

queuing model　排队模型

queuing system　排队系统

queuing theory　排队论

quota management　定额管理

quota reserve of medical supplies　药材储备定额

R

radiation accident　放射事故

radioactive pollution　放射性污染

radioactive sewage　放射性污水

radiographer　放射科技师

radiologist　放射科医师

radiology　放射学

random effect　随机效应

random effect model　随机效应模型

random error　随机误差

random sampling　随机抽样

random simulation　随机模拟

random variable　随机变量

randomization　随机化

randomized blind controlled clinical
　trial　随机盲法对照临床试验

randomized block design　随机区组
　设计

randomized consent design　随机应
　从设计

randomized controlled trial　随机对
　照试验

randomized parallel control trial
　随机平行对照试验

range　范围;区域;极差

rank correlation　秩相关

rank order　秩次

rank reviewing　等级评审

ranked data　等级资料

ranking method　排列法

rank-order stability analysis（ROSA）
　排序稳定性分析方法

rate　率

rate of successfully saving emergent
　patients　急诊抢救成功率

rate of time preference　时间偏好率

rating scale method　评定量表法

rating scales　等级评分法

rating scales method　业绩评定表

ratio scale scores　比值尺度分值

rational configuration　合理配置

rational decision making　理性决策

rational distribution　合理布局

rational drug use　合理用药

rational expectations　理性预期

rational use of medicines　合理用药

rationality　理性

reaction function　反应函数

real interest rate　实际利率

rear area　后方区

rear hospital　后方医院

reassurance value　放心价值

receiver operator characteristic curve
受试者工作特征曲线

reception triage　收容分类

receptivity；the level of acceptance
接受程度

recheck　复核

reciprocity　互利

recognition and approval
arrangement　承认和批准协议

record　记录

record of labor-hours lost　误工记录

records from management review
管理评审记录

recovery　恢复

recruit　招聘

recurrent cost　经常性开支成本

Red Cross Society（RCS）　红十字会

redeem；compensation　补偿

reevaluation　重新评价

reference concentration　参考浓度

reference dose　参考剂量

reference instructions　参照细则

reference price system　参考定价
体系

reference pricing of drugs　药品参
考定价

reference range　参考值范围

reference standard　参照标准

reference standard of diagnosis　诊
断参照标准

references test bias　参考试验偏倚

referral center　转诊中心

reform　改革

reform in economic structure　经济
结构改革

reform of government institutions
政府机构改革

reform of medical insurance system
医疗保险制度改革

reform of rural taxes and
administrative charges　农村税费
改革

reform of the urban housing system
城镇住房制度改革

regiment or brigrade aid station　团
（旅）救护所

regimental aid station　团救护所

region　区域

regional health planning　区域卫生

规划

regional rescue   区域性救治

register；registration   登记

registration fee   挂号费

registration office   挂号处；挂号室

regression   回归

regression forecasting model   回归
预测模型

regular education   正规教育

regular storage   经常性储备

regulation   规章

regulation economics   调控经济学

rehabilitation   康复

rehabilitation counseling   康复咨
询学

rehabilitation nursing   康复护理学

rehabilitation sanatorium care   康复
疗养

rehabilitation therapy   康复治疗

reimbursement   补偿

reimbursement list of drugs   报销药
品目录

reinforcement theory   强化理论

reinsurance company   再保险公司

rejuvenation of population   人口年
轻化

relapse   复发

relational model   关系模型

relative factor forecasting method
相关因素预测

relative legal problem   相关法律
问题

relative price   相对价格

relative risk   相对危险度

relay hospital   中转医院

reliability   可靠性；信度

renal transplant（RT）   肾脏移植

renew   续保

renewal of contract   续约

rent   租赁

rent expense，rent   租金支出

rent revenue/income   租金收入

rent seeking   寻租

repair and maintenance cost   修
缮费

repeatability；reproducibility   可重
复性

repeated cross-sectional surveys   重
复横断面调查

repeated follow-up study   重复随访
研究

repeated measure study   重复测量
研究

repeated measurement data   重复测

量资料

repeated survey　重复调查

replacement cost　替代成本法

report punctually　按时报告

report system　报告制度

reporter gene　报告基因

reporting bias　报告偏倚

reproducibility　重复性

reproductive health　生殖保健

reproductive ratio　复现率

reputation　声誉

rescue group of company　连抢救组

research & development　研发

research institute　研究所

research papers　研究论文

reserve fund　准备金

reserve of health service units　卫勤
　预备力量

reserve of medical supplies　药材
　储备

resident physician　住院医师

residential building　住宅

residual　残差

residual rights of claim　剩余索取权

residual rights of control　剩余控
　制权

resistance　抵抗力;抗(药)性

resource　资源

resource allocation　资源配置

resource based relative value system
　（RBRVs）　以资源为基础的相对价
　值标准

resource efficiency　资源效率

resource management　资源管理

resource scarcity　资源稀缺

respondent　被调查者

response　反应

responsibility　责任；职责

responsiveness　反应性

responsiveness assessment of patients
　患者反应性评估

rest home　休养所

restraint　约束

restrict　制约

resuscitation room　抢救室

retail of drugs　药品零售

retiring cadre office　离退休干部局

retrieval　检索

retrospective analysis　回顾性分析

retrospective cohort study　回顾性
　队列研究

retrospective study　回顾性研究

return on investment　投资回报

return visit　复诊

returns;reward   报酬

revealed/observed preference study   显示偏好法

revenue   收益

revenue curve   收益曲线

revenue function   收益函数

revenue maximization   收益最大化

review   审查；评审

reward   薪酬

right   权利

rights of a patient   患者的权利

rights of free contracting   自由签约权

rights of use   使用权

rights to share   收益权

rigidity   刚性

risk   风险；危险

risk acceptance   风险承担

risk adjustment   风险调整

risk analysis   风险分析

risk and cost   风险和成本

risk averse   风险厌恶

risk avoidance   风险回避

risk behavior   危险行为

risk coefficient   风险系数

risk control   风险控制

risk factor   危险因素

risk function   风险函数

risk ratio   危险度

risk selection   风险选择

risk transfer   风险转移

rival   竞争对手

Rosser index   罗素指数

rotating renewal of medical supplies   药材轮换更新

round   巡诊

route of transmission   传播途径

routine decision   常规决策

routine inspection   例行检验

routine reserve of medical supplies   药材日常储备

rule   规则

rule and regime of medical care   医疗规章制度

rule of diminishing return   报酬递减规律

rules and regulations   规章制度

rules for quality evaluation   质量评定规则

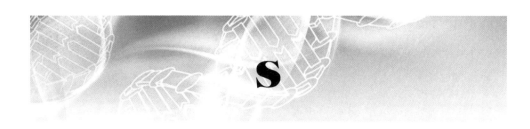

S

safeguard；ensure　保障

safety certification　安全认证

safety management　安全管理

safety responsibility system　安全责任制

safety stock　安全库存

sales price　销售价格

sales profit　销售利润

sales revenue　销货收入

sales volume　销售量

salvage　抢救

sample　样本

sampling　抽样

sampling error　抽样误差

sampling inspection　抽样检验

sampling quality supervision　抽样质量监督

sampling survey　抽样调查

sanatorium　疗养院

sanitarian office　保健局

sanitary and anti-epidemic administrative division　卫生防疫局

sanitary and anti-epidemic detachment　卫生防疫队

sanitary and anti-epidemic division　卫生防疫处

sanitary and anti-epidemic element　卫生防疫所

sanitary and anti-epidemic laboratory team　卫生防疫检验所

sanitary and anti-epidemic reconnaissance　卫生防疫侦察

sanitary Supervision Office　卫生监督办公室

satisfaction　满意；满足

satisfactory level of clinical service　临床服务满意度

Savings-type social insurance　储蓄性社会保险

scale of capital operation　资本运营规模

scarcity　稀缺性

scatter plot　散点图

scheme　方案

school of objective strategy　目标战

略学派

scientific forecasting　科学预测

scientific knowledge　科学知识

scientific management　科学管理

scientific research achievement
　　appraisal　科学成果鉴定

Scientific Research and Training
　　Division　科技训练局

scope effect　范畴效应

scope of medical aid　救治范围

scrapping criteria of medical supplies
　　药材报废标准

scrapping of medical supplies　药材
　　报废

screening　筛选

search strategy　检索策略

season storage　季节性储备

seasonal alteration forecasting
　　method　季节变动预测法

seasonal worker　临时工

second best theory　次优理论

second line hospital　二线医院

second party inspection　第二方检验

secondary environment　次生环境

secondary pollutants　二次污染物

secondary prevention　二级预防

secondary research evidence　二次

研究证据

secondary study　二次研究

second-class hospital at grade 1　一
　　级乙等医院

second-class hospital at grade 2　二
　　级乙等医院

second-class hospital at grade 3　三
　　级乙等医院

section chief　科长

section director　科主任

section of pharmaceutical
　　preparation　药剂科

sector hospital　部门所属医院

security control; security supervision
　　安全监管

security needs　安全的需要

security precaution　安全防范

security protection　安全保护

select　遴选

selection bias　选择性偏倚

self aid　自救

self control　自我控制法

self development　自我发展

self health care　自我保健

self-accumulation　自我积累

self-actualization　自我实现

self-control　自控

self-criticism　自我批评

self-employed　个体经济

self-esteem need　自尊的需要

self-initiative　自发

selfish departmentalism　本位主义

self-organization　自体组织

self-payment fee　自费

self-protect consciousness　自我保护意识

self-restraint　自我约束

self-sufficiency　自给自足

semi fixed cost　半固定成本

semi variable cost　半变动成本

semi-logarithmic line graph　半对数线图

semi-parametric model　半参数模型

senior engineer　高级工程师

senior human resources　高级人力资源

sensitivity　灵敏度

sensitivity analysis　敏感性分析

separate medical detachment　独立医疗队

separate medicine and authority　医政分离

sequela　后遗症

sequential decision　序贯决策

sequential design　序贯设计

sequential trial　序贯试验

serializing　系列化

service　服务

service costs　服务成本

service oriented management　服务型管理

service quality　服务品质

service remedy theory　服务补救理论

service revenue　服务收入

service supervision　服务监督

serving population　服务人群

settlement of accident；accident disposal　事故处理

severely wounded ward　重伤室

severity of wound　伤势

sewage discharge　污水排放量

sewage treatment　污水处理

sewage treatment equipment　污水处理设备

sex ratio　性别比率

shadow price of capital　资本影子价格

share of health expenditure in different population　不同人群所担负医疗费用

shift of aid station　救护所转移

ship medical department　舰艇卫生部门

shortage　短缺

shortcut　捷径

short-run marginal cost　短期边际成本

short-run total cost　短期总成本

short-term borrowings/debt　短期借款

short-term cost curve　短期成本曲线

short-term forecast　短期预测

short-term investment　短期投资

short-term orientation　短期导向

short-term planning　短期规划

short-term supply curve　短期供给曲线

shrinkage　缩减率

sick leave　病假

sickness impact profile　疾病影响量表

sickness insurance　疾病保险

similar approach degree　相似接近度

simple randomization　简单随机化

simulated cost　模拟成本

simulating forecast　模拟预测

single blind　单盲

single-payer plan　单一支付者计划

situational analysis　现况分析

size of the organization　组织规模

skill analysis　技能分析

skin temperature　皮肤温度

social and behavioral pharmacy　社会行为药学

social assistance system　社会救助体系

social benefit　社会效益

social burdens　社会负担

social capital　社会资本

social commonweal organization　社会公益机构

social contact need　社交的需要

social cost　社会成本

social drinking　社交性饮酒

social gambling　社交性赌博

social health strategy　社会卫生策略

social insurance　社会保险

social interaction　社会相互影响

social investigation method　社会调查法

social joint relief　社会共济

social medical insurance　社会医疗保险

social medicine   社会医学

social order   社会秩序

social pharmacy   社会药学

social psychology   社会心理学

social public relations   社会公共关系

social responsibility   社会责任

social security   社会保障

social security institution   社会保险机构

social security system   社会保障体系

social service   社会服务

social stabilizer   社会稳定器

social support   社会支持

social unified raising and personal account system   社会统筹与个人账户结合的模式

social welfare   社会福利

social welfare fund   社会福利金

social welfare home   社会福利院

socialization   社会化

socialization of hospital logistics service   医院后勤服务社会化

societal benefit   社会效益

Society for Medical Decision Making   医疗决策制定协会

society supervision   社会监督

socioeconomic evaluation of drug therapy   药物治疗的社会经济评价

soft science   软科学

soil contamination   土壤污染

solid waste   固体废弃物

source-oriented medical record   数据源定向的病历

spatial effect；spatial validity   空间效力

special medical fee   特定医疗费

special right to intervene   特殊干预权

specialist   专家

specialist care   专科护理

specialist hospital   专科医院

specialist-scored method   专家评分法

specialization   专业化

specialized medical centre   医学专科中心

specialized skill   业务专长

specialized treatment   专科治疗

specialty of Chinese medicine   中医专业

specialty of epidemic prevention   卫生防疫专业

specialty of lab test　检验专业

specialty of nuclear medicine　核医
学专业

specialty of pathology　病理专业

specialty of physical therapy　理疗
专业

specialty of radiation　放射专业

specialty of stomatology　口腔专业

specificity　特异度

spectrum bias　疾病谱偏倚

spectrum of disease　疾病谱

spectrum of health effect　健康效
应谱

speech therapist　言语治疗师(士)

sphere of application　适用范围

spiritual needs　精神需要

spontaneous investment　自发投资

stability　稳定性

staff　职工

staffing　人事

stakeholder　利益相关者

standard　标准

standard control　标准对照

standard cost system　标准成本体系

standard deviation　标准差

standard drug　标准药物

standard error of mean　均数的标
准误

standard examination for approval
标准报批审查

standard gamble　标准博弈法

standard grading　标准分级

standard medical cost　标准医疗
成本

standard of living　生活标准

standard of medical supply　药材补
给标准

standard substance　标准物质

standard system　标准体系

standardization　规范化;标准化

standardization management　标准
化管理

standardization of military medical
supplies　军用药材标准化

standardization principle　标准化
原则

standardize the tax system　规范
税制

standardized administration　标准化
管理

standardized allocation　标准配置

standardized bankruptcy procedures
规范破产

standardized cost-accounting system

标准成本核算系统

standardized management in sickroom　病室规格化管理

standardized mean difference　标准化均数差

standardized medical cost　标准医疗成本

standardized method　标准化法

standardized mortality rate　标准死亡率

standardized mortality ratio（SMR）标化死亡率比

standardized rate ratio（SRR）标化率比

standards program　标准规划

standing medical supplies in wartime　战时常备药材

standing plans　长效性计划

star-nursing　星级护理

State Administration of Traditional Chinese Medicine　国家中医药管理局

state basic medical insurance　国家基本医疗保险

State Bureau of Commodity Prices　国家物价局

state controlling　国家控股

State Development Planning Commission　国家发展计划委员会

State Economic and Trade Commission　国家经济贸易委员会

State of Food and Drug Administration（SFDA）国家食品药品监督管理局

state holding　国家持股

stated preference　陈述偏好

state-owned　国有

state-owned and private management model　国有和民营管理模式

state-owned capital　国有资本

state-owned enterprises　国有企业

state-owned share　国家股

state-type social insurance　国家型社会保险

statistical analysis　统计分析

statistical analysis of customer satisfaction　顾客满意度统计分析

statistical decision　统计型决策

statistical graph　统计图

statistical induction　统计归纳

statistical information　统计信息

statistical survey　统计调查

statistical table　统计表

statistical testing　统计试验

statistics   统计

statutory   法定

Steering Office of Medical
　　Department of CPLA   全军保健
　　领导小组办公室

sterile supply centre   消毒供应中心

sterilization   灭菌

sterilization and medical supply room
　　消毒供应室

stimulants   兴奋剂

stimulation compatibility   激励相
　　容性

stochastic double blind controlled
　　experiment   随机双盲对照试验

stochastic model   随机模型

stock amount of medical supplies
　　药材库存量

stock right   股权

stockholder   股东

storage costs   储存成本

storage fixed costs   固定储存成本

storage model   存储模型

storage of medical supplies   药材
　　保管

store room   储藏室

store-house for medical supplies   药
　　材库房

strategic cooperation   战略协作

strategic decision   战略决策

strategic guideline   战略方针

strategic objective   战略目标

strategic rear   战略后方

strategic reserve of medical supplies
　　药材战略储备

strategy   战略

strategy control   战略控制

strategy deployment   战略部署

strategy implementation   战略实施

strategy implementation effect   战
　　略实施效果

strategy implementation system   战
　　略实施体系

strategy management   战略管理

strategy management model   战略管
　　理模型

strategy planning   战略规划

stratification   分层

stratified random sampling   分层随
　　机抽样

stratified randomization   分层随
　　机化

stratified sampling   分层抽样

street hospital   街道医院

strength   强势

strength-opportunity strategy　优势-机会战略

strength-threat strategy　优势-威胁战略

structure and form　格局

structured problems　结构性问题

subclinical infection　亚临床感染；无症状性感染

sub-cohort study　亚队列研究

sub-committee　分委员会

subconscious　潜意识

subgroup analysis　亚组分析

subject construction；discipline construction　学科建设

subjection rapport；relationship of administrative subordination　隶属关系

subjective expected utility　主观预期效用

subsidy　津贴

subsistence allowances　最低生活保障

subsistence allowances for laid-off workers　下岗职工基本生活费

substantive system　实体系统

substitutes　替代品

substitution effect　替代效应

substitution parameter　替代参数

success rate in rescuing　抢救成功率

sufficient condition　充分条件

suitability　适应性

summary　汇总

superintend department　主管部门

supervise　监督

supervisor　主管人员

supervision of medical insurance　医疗保险监督

supplementary major expense insurance　补充大额医疗费

supplementary medical insurance　补充医疗保险

supply　供给

supply curve　供给曲线

supply function　供给函数

supply room　供应室

supply shock　供给冲击

supply system　供给系统

support system　支持系统

supportive leadership　支持型领导

surfactant　表面活性剂

surgeon　外科医师

surgical nursing　外科护理学

surgical ward　外科病房

surplus　盈余

surplus rural workers　农村剩余劳动力

survival analysis　生存分析

survival check　生存检验

survival crisis of hospital　医院生存危机

survival curves　生存曲线

survival function　生存函数

survival of the fittest　优胜劣汰

survival rate　生存率

survival time　生存时间

susceptibility　易感性

susceptible population　易感人群

sustainable development　可持续发展

SWOT analysis　SWOT 分析法

symmetry of information　信息对称

symptom　症状

synergism　增强作用

synergy effect　协同效应

system analysis　系统分析

system engineering　系统工程

system environment　系统环境

system evaluation　系统评价

system innovation　制度创新

system level　系统层次

system management　系统管理

system method　系统方法

system model　系统模型

system network architecture　系统结构

system of appointing　任命制

system of cooperative medical care　合作医疗体系

system of job responsibility in management by objectives　医院后勤服务目标管理责任制

system of medical supply　药材供应体制

system of president in charge　院长负责制

system of subsistence allowances　最低生活保障制度

system optimization　系统优化

system performance　系统绩效

system reform　体制改革

system science　系统科学

system thought　系统思想

systematic error　系统误差

systematic sampling　系统抽样

systematic thinking　系统思考

systematics　系统论

systemic efficiency　系统效率

T

tactical decision　战术决策

tactical rear　战术后方

tactical reserve of medical supplies
　药材战术储备

tactics　战术

take a risk　承担风险

talents　人才

tangible assets　有形资产

target control　目标控制

target decomposition　目标分解

target expansion　目标展开

target management elements　目标
　管理要素

target monitoring　目标监测

target principle　目标原则

target stimulation　目标激励

target structure　目标结构

target；objective；goals　目标

task of medical aid　救治任务

task preparation　任务准备

tax rate　税收率

tax-for-fees reform　费改税改革

tax-free service　免税服务

teaching and research section of
　pharmacy　药学教研室

teaching assistant　助教

teaching hospital　教学医院

team building　团队建设

team learning　团队学习

technical agreement　技术协议书

technical appraisals of malpractice
　医疗事故技术鉴定

technical appraisement　技术鉴定

technical cooperation　技术合作

technical decision　技术决策

technical duty　技术职务

technical efficiency　技术效率

technical management　技术管理

technical management board　技术
　管理委员会

technical properties　技术特性

technical standard of military
　medical　军用药材技术标准

technical-economic index　技术经济
　指标

technician　技士；技术员

technician; technologist   技术人员

technological knowledge   技术知识

technological progress   技术进步

technological specification   技术
规范

technologist   技师；技术专家

technologist-in-charge   主管技师

technology   技术

technology assessment   技术评估

technology evaluation   技术评价

technology resources   技术资源

technology service   技术服务

technology support   技术支撑

technology transfer   技术转让

temporary payments   暂付款

temporary receipts   暂收款

tendency; trend   趋势

terminal quality   终末质量

termination of insurance relations
保险关系终止

termination of risk   保险责任终止

tertiary prevention   三级预防

test   检验；试验

test for homogeneity   齐性检验

test of goodness   拟合优度检验

test report   测试报告；检验报告

tests for heterogeneity   异质性检验

tests for homogeneity   同质性检验

the content of financial management
财务管理内容

the core of hospital culture   医院文
化的核心

the correlation tree method   关联
树法

the cost of epidemic prevention   卫
生防疫费

the cost of family planning   计划生
育费

the cost of medical goods   卫生材
料费

the decision theory approach   决策
理论法

the depreciation charge of fixed
capital   固定资产折旧费

the entanglement between patients
and nurses   护患纠纷

the functions of financial
management   财务管理职能

the group behavior approach   集体
行为法

the influence of hospital culture   医
院文化影响

the information of diagnosis and
treatment   诊疗信息

the interpersonal behavior approach
人际行为法

the level of responsiveness of health
system　卫生系统的反应水平

the limit of authority or power
权限

the management of medical waste
医疗废物管理

the method of social need
investigation　社会需求调查法

the operational approach　经营法

the price formation mechanism　价
格形成机制

the price of medical service　医疗服
务价格

the principle of financial
management　财务管理原则

the process of financial management
财务管理环节

the rate in good condition　完好率

the reform of medical system　医疗
体制改革

the responsiveness of health system
医疗系统反应性

the retirement pension system　养老
保障制度

the right of autonomy　自主权

the right of awareness　知情权

the right of health　健康权

the right of privacy　隐私权

the risk of medical obligation　医疗
责任风险

the risk of medical practice　医师职
业风险

the risk of medical technology　医
疗技术风险

the role of hospital culture　医院文
化的角色

the system of accreditation　认证
制度

the system of basic old-age insurance
for enterprise employees　企业职
工基本养老保险制度

the system of income distribution
收入分配制度

the transfer of rural surplus labors
农村剩余劳力的转移

the trend of development　发展趋势

theorem　定理

theoretical interpretation　理论解释

theoretical model　理论模型

theoretical profit　理论收益

theory of constraints（TOC）　约束
理论

theory of management decision　管理决策理论

therapeutic equipment　治疗设备

therapeutic fee　治疗费

therapeutic room　治疗室

therapeutics　治疗学

thinking　思维

thinking mode　思维模式

third party certification　第三方认证制度

third party inspection　第三方检验

third-class hospital at grade 1　一级丙等医院

third-class hospital at grade 2　二级丙等医院

third-class hospital at grade 3　三级丙等医院

threat　威胁

three grade nursing　三级护理

three-level quality control　三级质量控制

threshold analysis　阈值分析

tidal current　潮流

time effect bias　时间效应偏倚

time preference　时间偏好

time series forecasting　时间序列预测

time trade-off　时间权衡法

time value of money　货币的时间价值

timing　时序

total cost　总成本

total cost accounting of a hospital　医院总成本核算

total cost management system　全面成本管理系统

total expenditure　总支出

total fertility rate　总和生育率

total fixed cost　总固定成本

total health expenditure　卫生总费用可变成本

total product　总产量

total quality control（TQC）　全面质量控制

total quality management（TQM）　全程质量管理

total quota　编制限额

total responsiveness of health system　医疗系统总体反应性

total revenue　总收益

total utility　总效用

total variable cost　总可变成本

township enterprises　乡镇企业

toxic reaction　毒力反应

traceability   可追溯性

traditional economy   传统经济

traditional health insurance   传统健康保险

traditional medicine   传统医学

training   培训

training detachment for medical corpsmen   卫生员训练队

training expense   训练费

transaction costs   交易费用

transform   变革

transform administrative fees into taxes   费改税

transform/shift the government functions   转变政府职能

transformation   转化;转变

transformation of hospital culture   医院文化转化

transformation of operational system   转制

transfusion room   输液室

transition probability   转换概率

transmission equipment   传导设备

transportation equipment   运输设备

treatment triage   救治分类

trend extrapolation   趋势外推法

triage   伤病员分类

triage evacuation hospital   分类后送医院

triage group   分类组

triage site   分类场

trusteeship model   托管模式

tuberculosis hospital   结核病医院

tumor hospital   肿瘤医院

turnover   人员流动

turnover rate of beds   病床周转率

two-way   二向

type approval   型式批准

type evaluation   型式评价

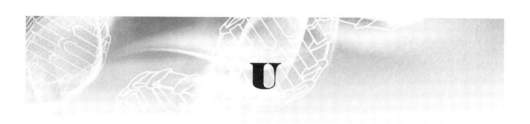

uncertainty　不确定性

unconditioned reflex　非条件反射

uncontrollable cost　不可控成本

underwriter　保险公司

underwriting agent　承保代理人

unemployment insurance　待业保险费

unemployment insurance benefits
　失业保险金

unfair competition　不公平竞争

unifying　统一化

unilateral arrangement　单边协议

unit hospital　队属医院

unit of measurement　测量单位

unit of work time　工时单位

unit value　单位值

United Nations Children's Emergency
　Fund（UNICEF）联合国儿童基金会

United Nations Development Programme
　（UNDP）联合国开发计划署

United Nations Fund for Population
　Activities（UNFPA）联合国人口
　基金会

universalization of military medical
　supplies　军用药材通用化

unpreventable risk　不可预防性风险

uranium poisoning　铀中毒

urban and rural residents with financial
　difficulties　城乡困难居民

urban housing provident fund　城镇
　住房公积金

urban social security system　城镇社
　会保障体系

urban subsistence allowance program
　城市最低生活保障

urbanization　城市化

urgent situation　紧急情况

urologist　泌尿科医师

utility　效用

utility function　效用函数

utility maximization　效用最大化

utility of drugs　药物效用

utility theory　效用理论

utilization　利用

utilization efficiency　使用效率

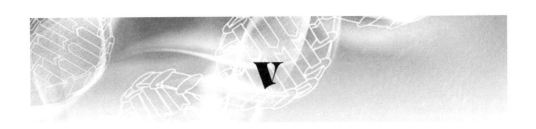

V

vacation　休假

vaccinate　接种

vaccine　疫苗

validation　确认

validity　真实性;效度

validity in time　时间效力

value　价值

value analysis　价值分析

value chain　价值链

value coefficient method　价值系
　数法

value engineering　价值工程

value engineering program　价值工
　程程序

value form　价值形态

value in health　健康价值

value maintaining　保值

value management　价值管理

value of information analysis　信息
　价值的分析

value of money　物有所值

value orientation　价值取向

value-based pricing　价值导向定价

variability　变异性

variable　变量

variable cost　变动成本;可变成本

variable cost　可变成本

variable input　可变投入

variance principle　方差原理

variation　变异

vector-cardiography room　心向
　量室

verifiability　可验证性

verifiable objective　可考核目标

verification　核实;验证

verification of conformity　合格
　证明

vertical equity　纵向公平

vertical relation　纵向联系

vertical transmission　纵向传播

vertical transportation　垂直运输

vested interests　既得利益

veterinary science　兽医学

vice commissar　副政委

vice dean in charge of medical
　services　业务副院长

vice director　副主任

vice minister　副部长

vice president　副院长

vicious cycle　恶性循环

vinculum　纽带

VIP waiting room　贵宾候诊室

virtual organization　虚拟企业

visiting students　进修生

visiting study　进修

vital index　生命指数

vital statistics　生命统计

vocational rehabilitation　职业康复

volume of medical care　医疗服务量

voluntary　自愿

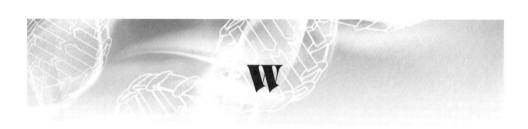

wage 工资

wage base 工资基数

wage bill 工资总额

wage criterion 工资标准

wage rate 工资率

wage system 工资制

wage-risk 工资-风险

waiting room 候诊室

want 要求

war internal medicine 野战内科学

war surgery 野战外科学

ward 病房

ward management 病房管理

ward of holding lightly wounded 轻伤留治室

ward organization 病区组织

washing room 洗涤室

weight 权重

weighted mean difference 加权均数差

weighted moving average forecasting method 加权移动平均预测法

welfare 福利

welfare economics 福利经济学

welfare organization 福利性机构

welfare-type social insurance 福利型社会保险

western medicine drugstore 西药房

whole course disaster management 全程灾备管理

whole life insurance 终身保险

willingness to accept（WTA） 意愿接受法

willingness to pay（WTP） 意愿支付法

wire communication 有线通信

wireless communication 无线通信

withdraw business license 吊销营业执照

withdrawal 退出

withdrawal symptoms 戒断症状

work diaries 工作日志法

work efficiency 工作效率

work environment 工作环境

work safety 劳动安全

workload 工作负荷

work-related injury   工伤

World Health Organization（WHO）

  世界卫生组织

wound condition   伤情

wound maker   伤标

wounded   伤员

wounded in action   战伤减员

wounded patient flow   伤员流

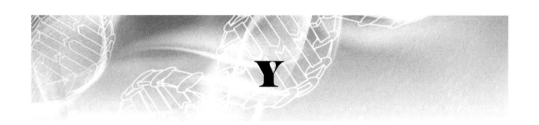

Y

years lived with disability　残疾挽救
生命年

years of life lost　死亡损失健康生
命年

years of life saved　挽救生命年

Youden's index　尤登指数

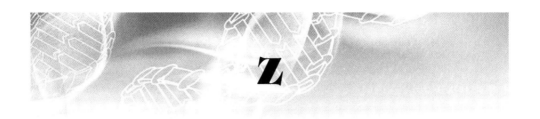

Z

zero cost　零成本

zero economic profit　零利润

zero elasticity　零弹性

zero population growth　人口零增长

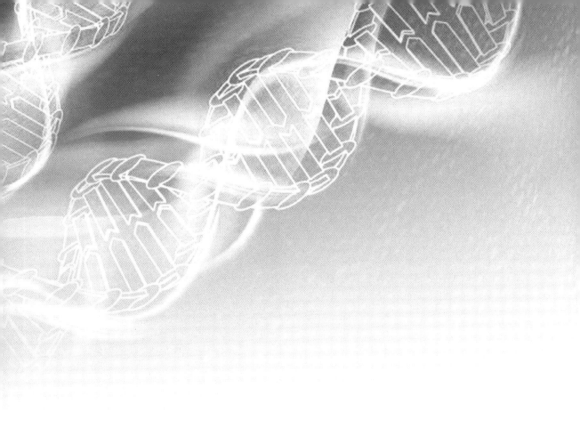

下 篇

中文—英文对照词汇

字母及其他

ABC 管理法　ABC management
method

B 超室　B-mode ultrasonic room

H 检验　H test

ISO 9001 标准　ISO 9001 standard

ISO 标准　ISO standard

PDCA 循环　plan，do，check，
action cycle

SWOT 分析法　SWOT analysis

Ⅰ期临床试验　phase Ⅰ clinical trial

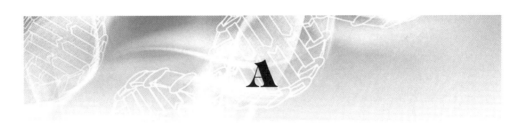

A

癌症患者生活功能指数 functional living index-cancer（FLIC）

癌症防治中心 cancer control and prevention center

安居乐业 live and work in peace and contentment

安乐死 euthanasia

安全保护 security protection

安全需要 security needs

安全防范 security precaution

安全管理 safety management

安全监管 security control；security supervision

安全库存 safety stock

安全认证 safety certification

安全认证标志 mark of safety certification

安全责任制 safety responsibility system

安慰剂 placebo

安慰剂效应 placebo effect

按服务付费 fee-for-service

按疾病诊断分类支付 diagnostic related groups（DRGs）

按劳分配 distribution according to work

按人头付费 capitation

按人头支付 per capita

按时报告 report punctually

按知分配 distribution according to knowledge

按资分配 distribution according to asset

案例法 case law

案例分析 case study

B

百分位数　percentile

半变动成本　semi variable cost

半参数模型　semi-parametric model

半对数线图　semi-logarithmic
　　line graph

半固定成本　semi fixed cost

半清洁区　half cleanness section

膀胱镜室　cystoscopy room

保管　preservation；storage

保健　health care

保健储蓄　medisave

保健基金　medifund

保健局　sanitarian office

保健科　department of health care

保健意识　health care consciousness

保健站　health station

保健中心　health care center

保健组织　health care organization

保险　insurance

保险标的物　object of insurance

保险储备　insurance storage

保险代理人　insurance agent

保险单　policy

保险范围　insurance coverage

保险方　insurer

保险费　premium

保险公司　insurance company

保险关系　insurance relations

保险关系终止　termination of
　　insurance relations

保险机制　insurance mechanism

保险基金　insurance fund

保险金　amount insured

保险经纪人　insurance broker

保险精算法　actuarial method

保险精算学　actuarial science

保险理赔　insurance claim

保险利益　insurable interest

保险赔付金额　compensation
　　pay-outs

保险评估　insurance evaluation

保险期　duration of insurance

保险期限　period of insurance

保险市场　insurance market

保险索赔　claim

保险统计　insurance statistics

保险要素　essence of insurance

保险业　insurance industry

保险义务　insurance obligation

保险因子　factor of insurance

保险责任　insurance liability

保险责任终止　termination of risk

保险总额,覆盖　coverage

保障　safeguard；ensure

保证金　guarantee fund

保证金;附属担保金

　　margins；collateral

保值　maintain value

报酬　returns；reward

报酬递减规律　rule of

　　diminishing return

报酬递增规律　increasing return

　　to scale

报告基因　reporter gene

报告偏倚　reporting bias

报告制度　report system

报销药品目录　reimbursement list

　　of drugs

暴发;流行　outbreak

暴露　exposure

暴露生物标志　biomarker

　　of exposure

贝叶斯公式　bayes' formula

贝叶斯方法　Bayesian method

备选方案　alternative project

备择假设　alternative hypothesis

背景问题　background questions

被保险方　insured

被调查者　respondent

被动管理　passive management

被服供应管理　clothing

　　supply management

被告　defendant

本一量一利分析　cost-volume-

　　profit analysis

本期损益　net income or loss for

　　current period

本位主义　selfish departmentalism

比较定价　comparision price system

比较优势　comparative advantage

比例　proportion；ratio

比例死亡比　proportional mortality

　　ratio（PMR）

比例研究　proportional or

　　proportionate study

比数;比值　odds

比值比　odds ratio

比值尺度分值　ratio scale scores

必需品　necessities

必要条件　necessary condition

边际成本　marginal cost

边际分析　marginal analysis

边际回报　marginal returns

边际生产率分配理论　distribution theory of marginal productivity

边际收益　marginal benefit

边际收益产品　marginal benefit product

边际收益递减规律　law of diminishing marginal return

边际替代递减　diminishing marginal substitution

边际替代率递减法则　law of diminishing marginal rate of substitution

边际效用　marginal utility

边际效用递减　diminishing marginal utility

边际效用递减法则　law of diminishing marginal utility

边际薪酬　marginal salaries

边际要素成本　marginal cost of factor

边界点　boundary point

边缘学科　frontier branches of science

编辑委员会　editing committee

编码　encoding

编制　authorized strength

编制限额　total quota

便利抽样　convenience sampling

便民服务　handy service for the public

变动成本;可变成本　variable cost

变革　transform

变量　variable

变异　variation

变异系数　coefficient of variation

变异性　variability

标化率比　standardized rate ratio（SRR）

标化死亡率比　standardized mortality ratio（SMR）

标准　standard

标准报批审查　standard examination for approval

标准博弈法　standard gamble

标准差　standard deviation

标准成本核算系统　standardized cost-accounting system

标准成本体系　standard cost system

标准对照　standard control

标准分级　standard grading

标准规划　standards program

标准化　standardization

标准化法　standardized method

标准化管理

　standardization management

标准化管理

　standardized administration

标准化均数差　standardized

　mean difference

标准化原则

　standardization principle

标准配置　standardized allocation

标准死亡率　standardized

　mortality rate

标准体系　standard system

标准文件　normative document

标准文件的应用　application of

　normative document

标准文件的制订　preparation of

　normative document

标准物质　standard substance

标准效度　criterion validity

标准药物　standard drug

标准医疗成本　standardized

　medical cost

标准转换　changing standard

标准总数　authorized amount

表面活性剂　surfactant

表面效度　face validity

饼图　pie chart

病案　medical record

病案计算机管理　computerized

　management of medical records

病案室　department of

　medical records

病床编设　determination of

　hospital beds

病床使用率　occupancy rate of

　hospitals beds

病床周转率　turnover rate of beds

病房　ward

病房管理　ward management

病假　sick leave

病理科　department of pathology

病理专业　specialty of pathology

病例　case

病例报告　case report

病例-对照研究　case-control study

病例管理　case management

病例讨论　case discussion

病区组织　ward organization

病室规格化管理　standardized

　management in sickroom

病死率　case fatality ratio

病因分值　etiologic fraction

病因学 aetiology

病种 category of diseases

病种医疗成本核算 disease-based cost accounting

病种质量控制 quality control of specified diseases

泊松分布 Poisson distribution

博弈 game

博弈论 game theory

补偿 redeem; compensation

补偿费 indemnity

补偿需求函数 compensated demand function

补偿原则 compensation principles

补充大额医疗费 supplementary major expense insurance

补充医疗保险 supplementary medical insurance

不定期检查 non-periodic inspection

不公平竞争 unfair competition

不合法、不合理资金筹集和收费 illegal and unjustifiable funds and charges

不可抗拒的因素 irresistible factors

不可控成本 uncontrollable cost

不可预防性风险 unpreventable risk

不良贷款 non- performing loans

不良反应 adverse reaction

不良事件 adverse event

不确定性 uncertainty

不适 discomfort; disorder

不同人群所担负医疗费用 share of health expenditure in different population

不完全成本 incomplete cost

不正常利润 abnormal profit

布局 disposition; layout

部长 minister; superintendent

部队医院 army hospital

部门 department

部门所属医院 sector hospital

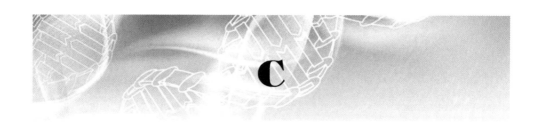

C

财务　finance

财务分析　financial analysis

财务风险　financial risk

财务管理对象　objects of financial management

财务管理环节　the process of financial management

财务管理环境　financial management environment

财务管理目标　financial management objectives

财务管理内容　the content of financial management

财务管理原则　the principle of financial management

财务管理职能　the functions of financial management

财务管理组织　organization of financial management

财务会计　financial accounting

财务活动　financial activities

财务计划　financial planning

财务监督　financial supervision

财务决策　account decision

财务科　financial affairs department

财务控制　financial control

财务实体　financial entity

财务影响　financial impact

财务预测　financial forecast

财务政策　financial policy

财务指标　financial index

财务制度　financial regulations

财务资本　financial assets

财政补贴基金　grant-in-aid fund

财政补助　financial subsidy

财政部　Ministry of Finance

财政偿还能力　ability to service debt

财政承受能力　financial capacity

财政管理　financial management

财政经济委员会　Finance and Economy Committee

财政收入　financial revenue

财政收支平衡原则　a principle of maintaining a balance between revenue and expenditures

财政支出　financial expenditure

采购 procurement

采购部门 department of purchasing

采购程序 procurement procedures

采购机制 mechanism of procurement

彩超室 color ultrasonic room

参保 proposal of insurance

参保单位 applicant unit

参保人 applicant

参考定价体系 reference price system

参考剂量 reference dose

参考浓度 reference concentration

参考试验偏倚 references test bias

参考值范围 reference range

参数 parameter

参数估计 estimation of parameter

参数检验 parametric test

参与型领导 participative leadership

参照标准 reference standard

参照细则 reference instructions

残差 residual

残疾 deformity；disability

残疾人 disabled person

残疾挽救生命年 years lived with disability

残留效应 carry-over effect

操作规程 agendum；operating instruction；operating manual

草案 draft

测量 measure

测量变异 measurement variation

测量单位 unit of measurement

测量的可行性 feasibility of measurement

测量控制体系 measurement control system

测量偏倚 measuring bias

测量评估者间信度 inter-rater reliability

测量评估者内信度 intra-rater reliability

测量误差 measurement error

测试报告；检验报告 test report

层次分析法 analytical hierarchy process

层次模型 hierarchical model

层次数据模型 hierarchical data model

查阅 look up；consult

差异化战略 differentiation strategy

产出最大化 output maximization

产房 delivery room

产科病房 maternity ward

产科医师　obstetrician

产品　product

产品安全　product security

产品性能报告　product performance report

产品质量　quality of products

产前检查室　pre-natal care room

产权　property right

产权关系　property right connection

产权收益　income from property

产业；行业　industry

产业布局　industrial layout；industrial distribution

产业结构　industry structure

长期边际成本　long-term marginal cost

长期不动产投资　long-term real estate in-vestments

长期导向　long term orientation

长期负债　long-term liabilities

长期股权投资　long-term equity investments

长期规划　long-term planning

长期借款　long-term loans payable

长期均衡　long-term equilibrium

长期平均成本　long-term average cost

长期失能　long-term disability

长期投资　long-term investments

长期预测　long term forecasting

长期预付租金　long-term prepaid rent

长期债券投资　long-term bond investments

长期总成本　long-term total cost

长效性计划　standing plans

肠镜室　enteroscopy room

肠胃病学　gastroenterology

偿付制度　payment system

常规决策　routine decision

常规武器减员　casualties caused by conventional weapons

常见病　common disease

常住人口　permanent population

超出法律范围　outside the law

超额利润　excess profit

超额赔款保险　excess of loss coverage

超声科　department of ultrasonography

超声心动图室　echocardiography room

潮流　tidal current

陈述偏好　stated preference

成本测算　cost accounting

成本递减　descending cost

成本递增法则　law of increasing cost

成本分析　cost analysis

成本函数　cost function

成本核算　cost accounting

成本结果分析　cost consequence analysis

成本竞争力　cost competitiveness

成本决算　financial account of cost

成本贴现值　precept value of cost （CPV）

成本效果　cost-effectiveness

成本效果比率　cost effectiveness ratio

成本效果分析　cost effectiveness analysis

成本效率　cost efficiency

成本效益比率　cost benefit ratio

成本效益分析　cost benefit analysis

成本效用比　cost utility ratio

成本效用比率　cost utility ratio

成本效用分析　cost utility analysis

成本预算　cost budget

成本中心　cost center

成本最小化　cost minimization

成果　achievement

成果应用　achievement application

成就取向型领导　achievement-oriented leader

承包经营　contractual operation

承保代理人　underwriting agent

承担风险　take a risk

承认和批准协议　recognition and approval arrangement

诚信　in good faith

城市"低保"　urban subsistence allowance program

城市化　urbanization

城乡困难居民　urban and rural residents with financial difficulties

城镇居民人均可支配收入　disposable income per capita in urban areas

城镇居民最低生活保障　a minimum standard of living for city residents

城镇社会保障体系　urban social security system

城镇职工基本医疗保险制度　basic medical insurance system for urban workers

城镇职工医疗保险制度改革　medical insurance reform in urban altd

城镇住房公积金　urban housing provident fund

城镇住房制度改革　reform of the urban housing system

乘积极限法　product-limited method

程序　procedure

程序化　programming

程序决策　programmed decision

迟报　delayed report

迟滞　hysteresis；retard

持续改进　continuous improvement

持续性学习　persisted learning

持续质量改进　continuous quality improvement

赤字预算　deficit budget

充分条件　sufficient condition

冲突　conflict

抽样　sampling

抽样调查　sampling survey

抽样检查百分比　percent sampling inspection

抽样检验　sampling inspection

抽样误差　sampling error

抽样质量监督　sampling quality supervision

筹划　plan and prepare

筹资的公平性　fairness of financial contribution

出厂价　producer price；manufacturer price

出口管理　export control

出口许可证制度　export license control

出勤　on duty

出生队列　birth cohort

出生率　birth rate

出院　discharge

出院患者数　number of separation

出院者人均医疗费用　average medical expense per inpatient

出资人；捐助者　contributor

出租资产　assets leased to others

初级抽样单位　primary sampling units

初级卫生保健　primary health care

初审　first hearing；first review

初始条件　initial condition

储藏室　store room

储存成本　storage costs

储蓄性社会保险　savings-type social insurance

处长　division chief

处方　prescription

处方药　prescription drugs

处置权　disposition right

传播途径　route of transmission

传导设备　transmission equipment

传递信息　pass information

传染　contagion

传染病　infectious disease；

　　contagious diseases

传染病报告　infectious

　　disease reporting

传染病监测　infectious

　　disease surveillance

传染病漏报率　percentage of

　　unreported infectious diseases

传染科　department of infection

传染源　infection source

传统健康保险　traditional

　　health insurance

传统经济　traditional economy

传统型医院　conventional hospital

传统医学　traditional medicine

床位需求量估算　estimation of

　　bed requirements

创伤外科　department

　　of traumatology

创新　innovation

创造力　originality；creativity

创造性思维　creative thinking

炊事设备　cooking equipment

垂直运输　vertical transportation

纯保险费　net premium

慈善事业　charities

次品　defective product

次生环境　secondary environment

次优理论　second best theory

粗出生率　crude birth rate

粗发病率　crude incidence rate

粗放管理　extensive management

粗放型发展模式　extensive

　　development model

粗死亡率　crude death rate

促进作用　promotion

存储模型　storage model

存货　inventories

存货短缺　critical stock position

存量　inventory

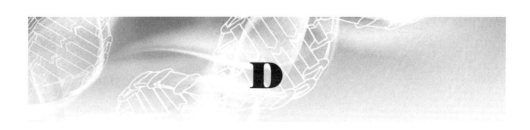

D

大局观念　overall perspective，
　overall views

大数法则　law of large number

大型医疗单位　large scale
　medical institution

代理处；机构　agency

待产室　labour room

待业保险费
　unemployment insurance

袋装处理　package treatment

单边协议　unilateral arrangement

单病种质量控制　disease-related
　quality control

单纯病例研究　case only study

单盲　single blind

单位值　unit value

单样本(组)t 检验　one sample/group
　t-test

单一价格法则　law of one price

单一支付者计划　single-payer plan

单因素方差分析　one
　factor ANOVA

导数　derivative

道德规范　moral norms

道德损害　moral hazard

德尔菲方法　Delphi method

德比克法则　De Bike Rules

德才兼备　have both ability and
　political integrity

登记　register；registration

登陆基地医院　base hospital
　at beachhead

等产量曲线　isoquant curve

等成本线　isocost line

等级评分法　rating scales

等级评审　rank reviewing

等级资料　ranked data

等利润曲线　isoprofit curve

等效　equivalence

低值易耗品　low-cost
　consuming products

抵抗力；抗(药)性　resistance

地方病　endemic

地方法院　district court

地理信息系统　geographic
　information system

地理因素 geographic factor

地区抽样 area sampling

地域管辖权 geographic jurisdiction

递增 progressive increase

第二方检验 second party inspection

第三方检验 third party inspection

第三方认证制度 third party certification

第一方检验 first party inspection

典型相关变量 canonical correlation variable

典型相关分析 canonical correlation analysis

典型相关系数 canonical correlation coefficient

点估计 point estimation

电子病历 electronic medical record

电子健康 E-health

电子商务 electronic commerce

电子数据交换 electronic data interchange

电子政务 electronic government

吊销 cancel；revoke；withdraw

吊销营业执照 withdraw business license

调查 investigation；investigate；inquire into

调查表 questionnaire

调查分析 investigation & analysis

调查者偏倚 interviewer bias

调控经济学 regulation economics

订货成本 purchase costs

定额管理 quota management

定价 pricing

定理 theorem

定量分析 quantitative analysis

定量目标 quantitative objective

定量预测 quantitative forecast

定量资料 quantitative data

定期检验 periodic inspection

定期支付形式 form of periodical payments

定时预测 periodical forecast

定性分析 qualitative analysis

定性决策 qualitative decision

定性目标 qualitative objective

董事会 directorate

动机 motive

动力设备 power equipment

动态分析 dynamic analysis

动态管理 dynamic management

动态规划 dynamic programming

动态监测 dynamic monitoring

动态模型 dynamic model

动态人群 dynamic population

动态组合　dynamic combination

动物毒素　animal toxin

动物实验　animal experiment

动物试验　animal trial

毒力反应　toxic reaction

独立核算　independent accounting

独立医疗队　separate
　　medical detachment

短期边际成本　short-run
　　marginal cost

短期成本曲线　short-term cost curve

短期导向　short-term orientation

短期供给曲线　short-term
　　supply curve

短期规划　short-term planning

短期借款　short-term borrowings
　　（debt）

短期投资　short-term investment

短期预测　short-term forecast

短期总成本　short-run total cost

短缺　shortage

队列　cohort

队列寿命表　cohort life table

队列效应　cohort effect

队列研究　cohort study

队列研究　cohort study

队属医院　unit hospital

对比　contrast

对策　countermeasure

对照　control

多边协议　multilateral arrangement

多层次系统　multi-level system

多次抽样　multiple sampling

多发病　frequently
　　encountered disease

多级抽样　multistage sampling

多目标决策　multi-objective decision

多向　multiway

多样性　diversity；multiplicity；
　　variety；versatility

多要素系统　multi-element system

多因子病　multifactorial disease

多元管辖权　diversity jurisdiction

多元线性回归　multiple
　　linear regression

多元协方差分析　analysis of
　　multiple covariance

多元性回归预测法　multivariate
　　regression forecasting method

多种所有制　diverse forms
　　of ownership

多重比较　multiple comparison

多重发表偏倚　multiple
　　publication bias

E

恶性循环　vicious cycle

恩格尔曲线　Engel curve

儿科　department of pediatrics

儿科门诊　outpatient department of pediatrics

儿科医师　pediatrician

儿科主任医师　professor of pediatrics

儿童外科　department of pediatric surgery

儿童医院　children's hospital

耳鼻喉科　department of otorhinolaryngology

耳鼻喉科医师　ear-nose-throat doctor

耳科学　otology

二次抽样　double sampling

二次检测法　double test method

二次污染物　secondary pollutants

二次研究　secondary study

二次研究证据　secondary research evidence

二级丙等医院　third-class hospital at grade 2

二级甲等医院　first-class hospital at grade 2

二级乙等医院　second-class hospital at grade 2

二级预防　secondary prevention

二审法院　court of second instance

二线医院　second line hospital

二向　two-way

二项式分布　binomial distribution

二重性　duality

F

发表偏倚　publication bias

发病率　incidence rate；morbidity

发病密度　incidence density

发明　invention

发展机会　development opportunity

发展计划　development plan

发展目标　development target

发展趋势　the trend of development

发展战略　developmental strategy

发作　attack

罚款　penalty；fine

法定　statutory

法令　decree

法律　law；legal

法律的实施　law enforcement

法律规范　legal norms

法律汇编　codification

法律监督　law supervision

法律委员会　law committee

法律责任　legal obligation

法人治理结构　corporate governance structure

法学　jurisprudence

法学家　jurist

法医学　forensic medicine

法院　court

反馈　feedback

反馈控制　feedback control

反馈频率　feedback frequency

反馈强度　feedback gain

反诉　counterclaim

反应　response

反应函数　reaction function

反应性　responsiveness

范畴效应　scope effect

范围；区域；极差　range

方案　scheme

方差分析　analysis of variance （ANOVA）

方差齐性　homogeneity of variance

方差齐性检验　homogeneity of variance test

方差原理　variance principle

方向性计划　directional plans

防护　protection；safeguard

防疫站　epidemic prevention station

146

防治措施 prevention and
treatment measures

放疗科 department of radiotherapy

放射防护 protection
against radiation

放射科 department of radiation

放射科技师 radiographer

放射科医师 radiologist

放射事故 radiation accident

放射性污染 radioactive pollution

放射性污水 radioactive sewage

放射学 radiology

放射专业 specialty of radiation

放心价值 reassurance value

非常规型决策 non-routine decision

非程序化决策 non-
procedural decision

非处方药 over-the-counter（OTC）

非传染性疾病 non-
infectious diseases

非对称性信息
asymmetric information

非经常营业损益 nonrecurring gain
or loss

非竞争性 noncompetitive

非均衡 disequilibrium

非确定型决策 decision

under uncertainty

非随机同期对照试验 non-
randomized concurrent
controlled trial

非条件反射 unconditioned reflex

非线性定价 nonlinear pricing

非线性回归预测法 nonlinear
regression forecasting method

非营利性 non-profit

非营利性机构 non-profitable agency

非营利组织 non-profit organization

非战斗减员 non battle casualties

非战斗外伤 non battle injury

非正规教育 irregular education

非正式计划 informal planning

非正式系统 informal system

非政府组织 non-governmental
organization（NGO）

废止 abolish

费改税 transform administrative
fees into taxes

费改税改革 tax-for-fees reform

费用分担 cost-sharing

费用分担的公平性 fairness in
financial contribution

费用管理 expense management

费用意识 cost consciousness

分布;分配　allocation

分布函数　distribution function

分布拟合　fitting of distribution

分层　stratification

分层抽样　stratified sampling

分层随机抽样　stratified
　　random sampling

分层随机化
　　stratified randomization

分化　differentiate

分级管理　hierarchical management

分级护理　graded nursing

分级救治　phased care

分类　classification

分类变量　categorical variable

分类标志　marker of triage

分类场　triage site

分类后送医院　triage
　　evacuation hospital

分类组　triage group

分立的产权　discrete property

分期偿还　amortization

分权　decentralization

分委员会　sub-committee

分支;分支机构　branch

分组变量　grouping variable

氛围　atmosphere

焚烧处理　burning treatment

焚烧炉　incinerator

风湿科　department of rheumatology

风险;危险　risk

风险承担　risk acceptance

风险调整　risk adjustment

风险分析　risk analysis

风险函数　risk function

风险和成本　risk and cost

风险回避　risk avoidance

风险控制　risk control

风险系数　risk coefficient

风险型决策　decision under risk

风险选择　risk selection

风险厌恶　risk averse

风险转移　risk transfer

封闭经济　closed economy

峰度　kurtosis

峰度系数　coefficient of kurtosis

服从　obedience

服务　service

服务补救理论　service
　　remedy theory

服务成本　service costs

服务观念　philosophy of service

服务监督　service supervision

服务经营型管理　operational model

of service management

服务品质 service quality

服务人群 serving population

服务收入 service revenue

服务型管理 service oriented management

服务质量 quality of service

弗里德曼检验 Friedman test

符合要求 conform requirements

福利 welfare

福利经济学 welfare economics

福利型社会保险 welfare-type social insurance

福利性机构 welfare organization

抚慰 appease

辅导者 counselor；mentor

辅助功能 auxiliary function

辅助决策 assistant decision-making

辅助设备 assistant equipment

辅助诊疗部门 assistant diagnosis and treat department

妇产科 obstetrics and gynecology department

妇科医师 gynecologist

妇科主治医师 gynecologist-in-charge

妇幼保健 maternal and child health

（MCH）

负二项式分布 negative binomial distribution

负反馈 negative feedback

负债 debt

附加保险费 additional premium

复发 relapse

复合泊松 compound Poisson

复合型 mixed mode

复合性 complex

复核 recheck

复现率 reproductive ratio

复相关系数 multiple correlation coefficient

复员转业军人 demobilized armymen

复诊 return visit

副部长 vice minister

副产品 by-product

副处长 deputy director general

副护士长 deputy supervisor of nursing care

副教授 associate professor

副科长 deputy section chief

副院长 vice president

副政委 vice commissar

副主任 vice director

副主任科员 deputy chief section member

副主任药师 associate chief pharmacist

副主任医师 chief-deputy physician

副总护士长 deputy chief head nurse

覆盖率 coverage rate

G

改革　reform

改进　improvement

概率　probability

概率抽样　probability sampling

概念系统　concept system

干预　intervention

干预措施　interventional procedures

肝胆外科　department of hepatobiliary surgery

感染发病率　incidence of infection

感染控制　infection control

感染控制委员会　infection control committee

刚性　rigidity

岗位变动　post alteration

岗位分析　job analysis

肛肠外科　department of anus & intestine surgery

高层次　high level

高级法院　high court of justice

高级工程师　senior engineer

高级人力资源　senior human resources

高技术产业　high-tech industry

高斯分布　Gaussian distribution

高投入、高消耗　high input，high consuming

高危人群　persons at risk of exposure

高压氧舱治疗中心　hyperbaric oxygen therapy center

高原病　high altitude sickness

告知义务　obligation to inform

哥顿法　Gorton method

格局　structure and form

隔离　isolate；isolation

隔离病房　isolation ward

隔离消毒　isolation and disinfection

个案医疗评价　case review

个人储蓄保险　personal savings insurance

个人发展计划　individual development plan（IDP）

个人价值　personal worth

个人见解　individual opinion

个人利益　personal interest

个人临床专长 individual clinical expertise

个人所得税 personal income tax

个人效益 private benefit

个人修炼 individual cultivation

个人需求函数 individual demand function

个人需求曲线 individual demand curve

个人医疗账户 individual medical insurance account

个人医疗账户基金 fund in individual medical insurance account

个人愿景 individual vision

个人责任 personal responsibility

个人账户 personal account

个人支付 out of pocket

个人智慧 individual wisdom

个人主义 individualism

个体化 individualization

个体经济 self-employed

个性化服务 personalized service

工程师;工程技术人员 engineer

工伤 work-related injury

工伤保险 employment(work) injury insurance

工时 man-hour

工时测定法 measurement of work time

工时单位 unit of work time

工效学 ergonomics

工业经济 industrial economics

工业性氟病 occupational fluorosis

工资 wage

工资标准 wage criterion

工资风险 wage-risk

工资基数 wage base

工资率 wage rate

工资制 wage system

工资总额 wage bill

工作负荷 workload

工作环境 work environment

工作伙伴 partner

工作绩效评价 auditing work performance

工作倦怠 job burnout

工作日志法 work diaries

工作设计 job design

工作效率 work efficiency

公费医疗 public health service

公费医疗制度 government welfare insurance scheme

公共产品 public goods

公共场所卫生管理条例 management regulations on sanitation regulation at public places

公共关系 public relation

公共关系目标 public relation goal

公共关系意识 public relation consciousness

公共关系咨询 public relations consulting

公共管理模式 public administration model

公共回归系数 common regression coefficient

公共金融学 public finance

公共偏好 public preference

公共事务 public affairs

公共收益 public benefits

公共卫生 public health

公共卫生服务 public health services

公共卫生设备 commonality health equipment

公共卫生事业 public health undertaking

公共选择 public choice

公共选择理论 public choice theory

公共政策 public policy

公共资源 public resources

公关机构 PR agencies

公关意识 PR-minded

公开采购 open procurement

公开招标 open tender

公立医院 public hospital

公平竞争 equal competition

公平性 fairness；equity

公益性 commonweal

公用财产 common property

公有制 public ownership

公正性 impartiality；equity

公众分析 public analysis

公众个体心理 public individual psychology

公众环境 public environment

公众群体心理 public community psychology

公众行为 public behavior

公众舆论 public opinion

功能分析 functional analysis

功能价值法 functional value method

功能障碍 functional disturbance；functional impairment

供给 supply

供给冲击 supply shock

供给函数 supply function

供给价格弹性　price elasticity of supply

供给量变化　change in quantity supplied

供给曲线　supply curve

供给系统　supply system

供给要素　factor supply

供需法　law of demand and supply

供应室　supply room

共负保险　co-insurance

共同被告　co-defendant

共同分摊费用　co-payment

共同愿景　common vision

沟通　communication

购买　acquisition

购买力　purchasing power

购买者　purchaser

购置费　purchase cost

估计　estimation

古典经济学　classical economics

股东　stockholder

股份制　joint-stock system

股份制医院　joint-stock system hospital

股利收入　dividends income

股权　stock right

股息　dividend

骨科医学　osteopathic medicine

骨伤科　department of bone fracture

固定保费　fixed premium

固定成本　fixed cost

固定储存成本　storage fixed costs

固定队列　fixed cohort

固定批量法　fixed order quantity

固定投入　fixed input

固定效应　fixed effect

固定效应模型　fixed effect model

固定信息　fixed information

固定资本　fixed capital；fixed assets

固定资产折旧费　the depreciation charge of fixed capital

固体废弃物　solid waste

顾客　customer

顾客财产　customer property

顾客财产控制程序　control procedure for customer property

顾客导向　customer oriented

顾客反馈　customer feedback

顾客服务　customer service

顾客服务联系表　customer service contact form

顾客沟通　customer communication

顾客价值链　customer's value chain

顾客满意　customer satisfaction

顾客满意度统计分析 statistical analysis of customer satisfaction

顾客投诉 customer complaint

顾客要求的识别 identification of customer requirements

雇员 employee

雇主 employer

挂号处；挂号室 registration office

挂号费 registration fee

拐点 inflection point

关键才能 core competency

关键控制点 critical control point

关键事件法 critical incident method

关节炎影响量表 arthritis impact measurement scale（AIMC）

关联 association

关联的一致性 consistency of the association

关联树法 the correlation tree method

关系模型 relational model

观察偏倚 observational bias

观察室 observation ward

观察性研究 observational study

观察研究 observational studies

观察终点 end point

官僚主义 bureaucracy

管道运输 pipeline transportation

管理地位 management position

管理方格图 managerial grid

管理费 administration cost

管理环境 managerial environment

管理会计 management accounting

管理价值观 management value concept

管理决策 managerial decision

管理决策理论 theory of management decision

管理流程 managing path

管理模式 management model

管理评审 management review

管理评审记录 records from management review

管理评审控制程序 management review control procedure

管理式医疗;管理型保健 managed care

管理视野 managerial perspective

管理体系 management system

管理效益 managerial benefit

管理信息系统 management information system

管理者代表 management representative

管理职能　management function

管理职责　management responsibility

贯彻；实施　carry out；implement

归类偏倚　misclassification bias

归纳法　induction

归因危险度　attributable risk

归因危险度百分比　attributable risk percent

归属　affiliation

归属的需要　affiliation needs

规范经济学　normative economics

规范破产　standardized bankruptcy procedures

规范税制　standardize the tax system

规范性预测　normative forecasting

规范研究　criterion research

规划　planning

规模报酬递减　descending returns to scale

规模报酬递增　increasing returns to scale

规模经济　economy of scale

规模收益不变　constant return to scale

规模收益递减　decreasing return to scale

规则　rule

规章　regulation

规章制度　rules and regulations

贵宾候诊室　VIP waiting room

国际标准　International Standard

国际标准的间接应用　indirect application of International Standard

国际标准的直接应用　direct application of International Standard

国际标准分类　classification of International Standard

国际标准化组织　International Standardization Organization（ISO）

国际合作　International Cooperation

国际疾病分类标准编码10　International Classification of Diseases 10（ICD-10）

国际水平标准　benchmark of International level

国际药物经济学与结果研究协会　International Society of Pharmacoeconomics and Outcomes Research

国际医疗质量协会　International Society for Quality in Health Care

（ISQHC）

国家持股　State holding

国家发展计划委员会　State Development Planning Commission

国家股　State-owned share

国家基本医疗保险　State Basic Medical Insurance

国家经济贸易委员会　State Economic and Trade Commission

国家控股　State controlling

国家食品药品监督管理局　State Food and Drug Administration

国家团体　National body

国家卫生服务　National Health Service（NHS）

国家卫生服务制度　National Health Service（NHS）System

国家物价局　State Bureau of Commodity Prices

国家型社会保险　State-type social insurance

国家药品政策体系　National Drugs Policies System

国家中医药管理局　State Administration of Traditional Chinese Medicine

国家临床标准研究所　National

Institute for Clinical Excellence （NICE）

国民待遇　national treatment

国民生产总值　gross national product

国民义务保险　national compulsory insurance

国务院办公厅　General Office of the State Council

国有　state-owned

国有和民营管理模式　state-owned and private management model

国有企业　state-owned enterprises

国有资本　state-owned capital

国有资产流失　loss of state assets

国有资产转化　National asset transformation

过程　process

过程控制　process control

过程评价　process evaluation

过程效用　process utility

过度供给　oversupply

过度生产能力定理　excess-capacity theorem

过度作用　over effect

过失　negligence；delinquency

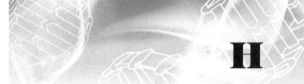

H

海军医院　navy hospital

函审　examination by letter

好转　improvement

合并方差　combined/
　pooled variance

合法的　legal

合法化　legitimatize

合法权益　legal interests

合法性　legality；legitimacy

合格保证　assurance of conformity

合格标志　mark of conformity

合格测试　conformity testing

合格品　qualified product

合格评定　conformity assessment

合格评定委员会　committee on
　conformity assessment

合格认证　conformity certification

合格认证标志　mark of
　conformity certification

合格证明　verification of conformity

合格证书　certificate of conformity

合理布局　rational distribution

合理配置　rational configuration

合理用药　rational drug use

合同　contract

合同制医师　contracted physician

合作联营模式　cooperate
　pooling model

合作医疗　cooperative health service

合作医疗体系　system of cooperative
　medical care

合作医疗制度　cooperative
　medical system

核磁共振　nuclear magnetic
　resonance（NMR）

核实　verification

核算　account

核心价值　core value

核心角色　key role；core role

核心竞争力　core competitiveness

核心领导　core leader

核心期刊　core journal

核心员工　core employee

核心职系　core grade

核医学科　department of
　nuclear medicine

核医学专业　specialty of

　nuclear medicine

黑箱方法　black box method

横断面研究　cross-sectional study

横向传播；水平传播

　horizontal transmission

横向公平　horizontal equity

横向联系　horizontal relation

红十字会　Red Cross Society（RC）

宏观调控　macro-control

宏观调控目标　macro-control targets

宏观管理　macro-management

宏观经济　macroeconomic

宏观经济模型

　macroeconomic model

宏观经济目标

　macroeconomic targets

宏观经济与健康委员会　Commission

　on Macroeconomics and Health

宏观决策　macro-decision

宏观配置　macro distribution

后方区　rear area

后方医院　rear hospital

后付制度　post payment

后勤　logistics

后勤保障部门　logistics department

后勤服务公司　logistics

service company

后勤管理　logistics management

后勤人事管理　Human resource

　management of

　logistics department

后勤设备管理　logistics

　equipment management

后勤物资供应　logistics

　material supply

后勤物资管理　logistics

　material management

后送分类　evacuation triage

后送适应证　indications

　for evacuation

后送文件袋　evacuation

　document envelope

后送医院　evacuation hospital

后遗症　sequela

候诊室　waiting room

呼吸科　department of

　respiratory medicine

互补品　complement goods

互救　buddy aid

互利　reciprocity

护患纠纷　the entanglement between

　patients and nurses

护理　nursing

护理安全　nursing safety

护理安全管理　nursing
safety management

护理标识　nursing mark

护理部　nursing department

护理部主任　director of
nursing department

护理成本　nursing cost

护理程序　nursing procedure

护理档案　nursing files

护理风险　nursing risk

护理风险处理　nursing risk handling

护理风险评价　nursing
risk evaluation

护理风险识别　nursing
risk identification

护理风险事件　nursing risk event

护理管理　nursing management

护理管理标准　nursing
management standard

护理管理技巧　nursing
management technique

护理管理体制　nursing
management system

护理管理者　nursing manager

护理过程　nursing processes

护理记录　nursing record

护理经济学　nursing economics

护理纠纷　nursing dispute

护理模式　nursing model

护理人力资源　nursing
human resources

护理人力资源管理　nursing human
resources management

护理人员配备　nursing human
resources allocation

护理任务　nursing task

护理信息学　nursing informatics

护理行为　nursing care activity

护理质量　nursing quality

护理质量评估　nursing
quality appraisal

护理资源　nursing resources

护理最小数据集　nursing minimum
data set

护师　nurse practitioner

护士　nurse

护士长　head nurse

护士站　nursing station

护士值班室　nurse's duty room

化疗　chemical therapy

化疗科　department
of chemotherapy

化学武器减员　casualties caused by

chemical weapons

化学性皮肤灼伤 chemical burns of skin

化学性眼部灼伤 chemical burns of eye

坏账转回利益 gain on reversal of bad debts

环节质量 process quality

环境保护 environmental protection

环境变量 environment variable

环境管理体系 environmental management system

环境监测 environmental monitoring

环境绿化 environment virescence

环境美化 environment beautification

环境匹配 matching environment

环境审核 environmental audit

环境卫生学 environmental hygiene

环境污染 environmental pollution

换药碗 dressing bowl

患病率 prevalence

患者 patient

患者的权利 rights of patient

患者的日常护理 daily care of patient

患者的义务 obligation of patient

患者第一 patients the first

患者反应性评估 responsiveness assessment of patients

患者分类 patient classification

患者管理 patient management

患者价值观 patient value perspective

患者利益 patient benefit

患者满意度 patient satisfaction

患者满意度评估 patient satisfaction appraisal

患者偏好 patient preference

患者预期事件发生率 patient's expected event rate

患者自报结果 patient-reported outcomes，PRO

黄金规则 golden rule

灰色关联度 grey relevancy degree

灰色文献 grey literature

恢复 recovery

回顾性队列研究 retrospective cohort study

回顾性分析 retrospective analysis

回顾性研究 retrospective study

回归 regression

回归系数 coefficient of regression

回归预测模型 regression

forecasting model

回扣　commission

汇总　summary

荟萃分析　Meta analysis

会诊　consultation

婚姻　marriage

混合成本　mixed cost

混合经济　mixed economy

混杂　confounding

混杂偏倚　confounding bias

混杂因素　confounding factor

混杂因子　confounder

豁免　exemption

豁免权　immunity

火线抢救　first aid in frontline

伙食费　diet fee

货币的时间价值　time value
　　of money

货币资本　currency capital

霍尔三维结构　Hall's three
　　dimensional structure

霍桑实验　Hawthorne experiment

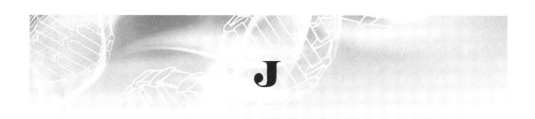

J

机关职能部门
administrative department

机会 opportunity

机会成本 opportunity cost

机遇节点 chance nodes

机制 machanism

机制调整 mechanism adjustment

肌电图室 electromyogram room

积极财政政策 a proactive
fiscal policy

积极的就业政策 a proactive
employment policy

基本分析 fundamental analysis

基本功能 basic function

基本结构 basic structure

基本理念 basic faith

基本能力 fundamental ability

基本权利 fundamental rights

基本生活费 basic living allowances

基本生命支持 basic life support

基本卫生服务 essential health
care services

基本协议 basic protocol

基本药品 essential drugs

基本医疗 basic medical care

基本医疗保险基金 funds of basic
medical insurance

基本医疗费用保险 basic medical
expense insurance

基本医疗服务 essential
medical service

基本原则 fundamental principle

基层监督 grass-roots supervision

基层卫生技术人才 health
technology man-power in
preliminary level

基层卫生监督 primary
health supervision

基层卫生与妇幼保健 primary health
and maternal & child health

基层预防保健网络 primary
preventive health care network

基础护理 basic nursing

基础理论成果 achievements in
basic theory

基础设施 infrastructure

基础研究 basic study

基础质量 basic quality

基地医院 base hospital

基金 funds

基金式 funding system

基年 base year

基线比较物 baseline comparator

基于疾病的模型 disease-based model

基准 benchmark

绩效 performance

绩效管理 performance management

绩效考核;绩效评估
performance appraisal

绩效评价 performance evaluation

绩效审查 performance review

激励 motivation

激励措施 motivation measures

激励机制 motivation mechanism

激励相容性
stimulation compatibility

激励因素 motivator

极大化 maximization

极端值 extreme value

极限分析 analysis of extremes

急救 emergency care

急救 first aid

急救医疗管理模式 emergency medical management model

急救医疗系统 emergency medical care system

急救医疗信息系统 emergency medical care information system

急救站 emergency service; first aid station（FAP）

急救中心 emergency center

急诊 emergency

急诊标准化管理 emergency standardization management

急诊程序化管理 emergency programmed management

急诊儿科 emergency pediatrics department

急诊费 emergency fee

急诊妇产科 emergency obstetrics and gynecology department

急诊观察室 emergency observation room

急诊化验室 emergency laboratory

急诊疾病谱 emergency disease spectrum

急诊监护室 emergency intensive care unit

急诊科 department of emergency

急诊内科　emergency internal
　medicine department

急诊抢救成功率　rate of successfully
　saving emergent patients

急诊人次数　person-time of
　emergency visits

急诊室　emergency room

急诊收费挂号　emergency
　registration & cashier office

急诊手术室　emergency
　operation room

急诊首诊负责制　emergency first-
　visit responsibility system

急诊外科　emergency
　surgery department

急诊药房　emergency pharmacy

急诊值班室　emergency duty room

急诊制度化管理　emergency
　institutionalized management

急诊治疗室　emergency
　therapeutic room

急诊自动传呼系统　automatic call
　system in emergency department

疾病　disease

疾病保险　sickness insurance

疾病成本　cost of illness

疾病成本估计　estimating the cost

of illness

疾病分布　distribution of disease

疾病分类　classification of diseases

疾病负担　burden of disease

疾病构成比　constituent ratio
　of disease

疾病监测　disease monitoring

疾病减员　casualties due to diseases

疾病控制中心　center of
　disease control

疾病谱　spectrum of disease

疾病谱偏倚　spectrum bias

疾病因果关系　disease causation

疾病影响量表　sickness
　impact profile

疾病预防控制局　Disease Defense
　and Command Office

疾病治疗成本　cost of therapy

疾病专用量表　disease
　specific instruments

集权　centralization of state power

集体股　collective shares

集体力量　collectivity power

集体目标　group objective；
　collective objective

集体思维　collective thinking

集体所有　collective ownership

集体行为法　the group
　　behavior approach

集体主义　collectivism

集体资本　collective capital

集约型模式　intensive
　　development model

集中采购　centralized procurement

集中管理　centralized management

集中趋势　central tendency

几何均数　geometric mean

计划财务处　planning and
　　financial division

计划管理　planning management

计划经济　planned economy

计划免疫　planed immunity

计划生育　family planning

计划生育费　the cost of
　　family planning

计划生育领导小组　Leading Group
　　of Birth Control

计量经济学　econometrics

计量模型分析　econometric
　　model analysis

计量确认　metrological confirmation

计量特性
　　metrological characteristic

计量资料　measurement data

计数资料　enumeration data

计算机辅助软件工程　computer
　　aided software engineering

计算机管理
　　computerized management

计算机模拟法　computerized
　　simulation method

计算机装备　computer equipment

记录　record

技能分析　skill analysis

技师　technologist

技士；技术员　technician

技术　technology

技术服务　technology service

技术管理　technical management

技术管理委员会　technical
　　management board

技术规范
　　technological specification

技术合作　technical cooperation

技术活动新领域　new field of
　　technical activity

技术鉴定　technical appraisement

技术进步　technological progress

技术经济指标　technical-
　　economic index

技术决策　technical decision

技术评估　technology assessment

技术评估办公室　office of
technology assessment

技术评价　technology evaluation

技术人员　technician；technologist

技术特性　technical properties

技术效率　technical efficiency

技术协议书　technical agreement

技术支撑　technology support

技术知识　technological knowledge

技术职务　technical duty

技术专家　technologist

技术转让　technology transfer

技术资源　technology resources

剂量-存活曲线　dose-survival curve

剂量-反应关系　dose-
response relationship

剂量效应　dose effect

剂量-效应曲线　dose-effect curve

季节变动预测法　seasonal alteration
forecasting method

季节性储备　season storage

既得利益　vested interests

继续教育　continuous education

继续医学教育　continuous
medical education

加拿大标准协会　Canadian

Standards Association

加拿大药物科学协会　Canadian
Society for Pharmaceutical
Sciences（CSPS）

加权均数差　weighted
mean difference

加权移动平均预测法　weighted
moving average
forecasting method

家庭　household；family

家庭（通科）医生　general physician

家庭病床　family sick-beds

家庭化护理　family-style nursing

家庭康复　family-
based rehabilitation

家庭医疗服务　home medical service

家庭医师　family doctor

家属医院　family hospital

家族（庭）聚集性
familial aggregation

家族（庭）聚集性研究　familial
aggregation study

家族（庭）相似性　family resemblance

价格　price

价格差别　price difference

价格弹性　price elasticity

价格调整模型　price

adjustment model

价格管制 price control

价格机制 pricing mechanism

价格理论 price theory

价格歧视 price discrimination

价格消费曲线 price
consumption curve

价格形成机制 the price
formation mechanism

价格指数 price index

价值 value

价值导向定价 value-based pricing

价值分析 value analysis

价值工程 value engineering

价值工程程序 value
engineering program

价值管理 value management

价值链 value chain

价值取向 value orientation

价值系数法 value
coefficient method

价值形态 value form

假定 assumption

假设 hypothesis

假设检验 hypothesis test

假设情境 hypothetical scenarios

假阳性率;误诊率 false positive rate

假阴性率;漏诊率 false negative rate

间接成本 indirect cost

间接法 indirect approach

间接护理 indirect nursing

间接经济负担 indirect burden

间接人工 indirect labor

间接融资手段 indirect
financing instrument

间接效益 indirect benefit

间接因果联系 indirect
causal association

兼并 merger

兼并重组 merger
and reorganization

监测;监控 monitoring

监督 supervise

监督员 supervisor

减压病 decompression sickness

减员 casualties

减员分析 analysis of casualties

减员增效 downsize staffs and
improve efficiency

检查费 physical examination fee

检查室 examination room

检查治疗室 examination &
therapeutic room

检索 retrieval

检索策略　search strategy

检验；试验　test

检验机构　inspection body

检验记录　inspection record

检验科　department of laboratory

检验效能　power of a test

检验专业　specialty of lab test

检疫　quarantine

检疫所　quarantine station

简单随机化　simple randomization

简略寿命表　abridged life table

建议成本　proposed cost

建筑密度　building density

健保双全　medishield

健康　health

健康保险　health insurance

健康保险制度　health
insurance system

健康测量指标　health measure

健康促进　health promotion

健康档案　health archive

健康风险指数　health risk index
（HRI）

健康福利计划　health benefits plan

健康公平性　equity in health

健康及意外险　health and
casualty insurance

健康价值　value in health

健康监视　health surveillance

健康检查　physical check-up

健康教育　health education

健康结果　health outcome

健康科学中心　health sciences center

健康领域模型　health field model

健康期望寿命　life expectancy

健康权　the right of health

健康损害　health lesion

健康投资　health investment

健康危险因素评价　health risk
factors appraisal（HRFA）

健康维持组织　health
maintenance organization

健康维持组织　health maintenance
organization（HMO）

健康相关生命质量　health-related
quality of life（HRQL）

健康效应谱　spectrum of
health effect

健康效用指数　health utility index

健康信息网络　health
information network

健康行为　health behavior

健康状况　health status

健康咨询　health consulting

舰艇卫生部门　ship medical department

渐进式改革　progressive reformation

鉴定　appraisal

鉴定过程　qualification process

讲师　lecturer

奖励制度　encouragement system

交叉补助　cross-subsidy

交叉感染　cross infection

交叉融合　cross integration

交叉设计　cross-over design

交叉试验　cross-over experiment

交互作用　interaction

交互作用归因比　attributable proportion of interaction

交易成本　deal cost；sanction cost

交易费用　transaction costs

交易流量　dealing flux

角度　perspective

矫形外科　department of orthopedics

矫形外科医师　orthopedist

教授　professor

教学科研　education and research

教学医院　teaching hospital

教育康复　educational rehabilitation

教育培训　education and training

接生员　midwife

接受程度　receptivity；the level of acceptance

接种　vaccinate

街道医院　street hospital

节育率（避孕率）　contraceptive prevalence rate

结构效度　construct validity

结构性问题　structured problems

结果　outcomes

结果节点　outcomes nodes

结果评价　outcome evaluation

结果研究　outcomes research

结合点　combining site

结核病　tuberculosis

结婚高峰　marriage boom

捷径　shortcut

截尾值　censored value

解剖学　anatomy

戒断症状　withdrawal symptoms

界定　identification

金标准　gold standard

金融资本　financial capital

金融资本运营　financial capital management

金融资产　finance asset

津贴　subsidy

紧急措施　emergency measure

紧急救治　emergency medical care

紧急情况　urgent situation

进城务工农民　migrant workers
　　in cities

进口许可证制度　import
　　license system

进入壁垒　entry barriers

进修　visiting study

进修生　visiting students

晋升　promotion

晋升考核　promotion assessment

经常性储备　regular storage

经常性开支成本　recurrent cost

经济　economy

经济成本　economic cost

经济定货量法　economic
　　order quantity

经济法规　economic regulation

经济福利　economic welfare

经济规模　economic scale

经济结构调整
　　economic restructuring

经济结构改革　reform in
　　economic structure

经济决策　economic decision

经济利润　economic profit

经济模型　economic model

经济适度快速增长　an appropriate
　　rapid economic growth

经济体系　economic system

经济效率　economic efficiency

经济效益　economic benefit

经济学　economics

经济学分析　economic analysis

经济学结果　economic outcomes

经济学评价　economic evaluation

经济周期　business cycle

经济租金　economic rent

经理　manager

经验法　empirical approach

经验事实　experimental fact

经验医学　empirical medicine

经营才能　operating ability

经营法　the operational approach

经营方式　business mode

经营管理　operation management

经营结构　management structure

经营预测　economic prediction

精确性　precision

精神变态者　psychopath

精神病科　department of psychiatry

精神病学专家　psychiatrist

精神病院　mental hospital

精神损害　mental impairment

精神需要　spiritual needs

精神依赖　psychological dependence

精神障碍　mental handicap

精神状态　mental state

精算师、保险统计员　actuary

净保费原理　net premium principle

净现值　net present value

净效益　net benefit（NB）

净需求　net demand

净资产　net asset

竞标法　bidding games

竞争　competition

竞争采购　competitive procurement

竞争对手　rival

竞争风险　competing risk

竞争力资源

　competitiveness resources

竞争聘任制度　competitive

　appointment system

竞争型决策　competitive decision

　making；decision under conflict

竞争性市场　competitive market

竞争性优势　competitive advantage

竞争性原则　competitive principle

竞争战略　competition strategy

纠错机制　error check mechanism

纠正措施　corrective action

酒精（乙醇）滥用　alcohol abuse

酒精依赖　alcoholism

救护车　ambulance

救护所　aid station

救护所配置地域　disposition district

　of aid station

救护所展开　aid station deployment

救护所转移　shift of aid station

救治范围　scope of medical aid

救治分类　treatment triage

救治任务　task of medical aid

救治种类　kinds of medical care

就业　employment

居家护理　home health care

举证责任　burden of proof

拒赔　claim rejected

聚集指数　cluster index

聚类分析　cluster analysis

决策　decision

决策层　decision-making layer

决策分析　decision analysis

决策过程　decision-making process

决策技术　decision technique

决策科学　decision science

决策理论法　the decision

　theory approach

决策论 decision theory

决策模式 decision model

决策目标 decision goal

决策树 decision tree

决策树分析 decision tree analysis

决策数学模型 mathematical model
of decision

决策学 decision-making study

决策原则 decision rule

决策支持系统 decision
support system

决定系数 coefficient
of determination

决定因素 determinant factor；
decisive factor

决定作用 decisive action

决算 final accounts

绝对优势 absolute advantage

军队卫生事业费 funds for military
medical service

军队卫生事业管理 military health
service administration

军队药材管理 military medical
supply administration

军队医院 military hospital

军事机构 military establishments

军事医学 military medicine

军事医学研究所 institute of
military medicine

军事医学院 military medical college

军医大学 military
medical university

军用药材标准化 standardization of
military medical supplies

军用药材技术标准 technical
standard of military medical

军用药材通用化 universalization of
military medical supplies

均方 mean square

均衡 equilibrium

均衡产量 equilibrium quantity

均衡发展 balanced development

均衡价格 equilibrium price

均衡条件 equilibrium condition

均数 mean

均数的标准误 standard error
of mean

均值原理 mean value principle

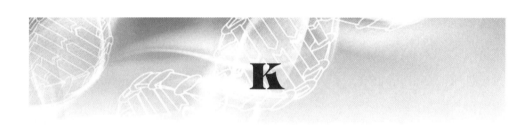

K

卡方分布　chi-square distribution

卡方检验　chi-square test

开放试验　open trial

康复　rehabilitation

康复护理学　rehabilitation nursing

康复疗养　rehabilitation
sanatorium care

康复医师　physiatrist；
rehabilitation physician

康复医院　convalescence hospital

康复治疗　rehabilitation therapy

康复咨询学
rehabilitation counseling

抗感染药物　anti-infection drugs

抗休组　antishock group

考克斯比例风险回归模型　Cox
proportional hazard regression

柯布-道格拉斯　Cobb-Douglas

柯布-道格拉斯生产函数　Cobb-
Douglas production function

科长　section chief

科副主任　deputy section director

科克伦图书馆　Cochrane library

科克伦系统评价　Cochrane
systematic review

科克伦协作网　Cochrane
collaboration network

科技教育司　Department of Science，
Technology and Education

科技训练局　Scientific Research and
Training Division

科室成本核算　departmental
cost accounting

科室主任　department chief

科学成果鉴定　scientific research
achievement appraisal

科学管理　scientific management

科学预测　scientific forecasting

科学知识　scientific knowledge

科主任　section director

可变成本　variable cost

可变投入　variable input

可承受性　affordability

可持续发展
sustainable development

可及性　accessibility

可接受性　acceptability

可考核目标　verifiable objective

可靠性;信度　reliability

可控成本　controllable cost

可控输入　controllable input

可信度　credibility

可信区间　confidence interval

可信限　confidence limit

可行性　feasibility

可行性研究　feasibility research

可验证性　verifiability

可重复性　repeatability;

　reproducibility

可追溯性　traceability

客观风险　objective risk

客观世界　objective world

客观证据　objective evidence

客户关系管理　customer

　relationship management

克鲁斯卡尔-沃利斯 H 检验　Kruskal-

　Wallis H test

空白对照　blank control

空间效力　spatial effect;

　spatial validity

空军医院　air force hospital

控制　control

控制变量　control variable

控制单位　control unit

控制对象　control object

控制过程　control process

控制技术　control technology

控制论　cybernetics

控制权　control right

控制手段　control methods

控制图　control chart

口腔/牙科科学　oral/dental sciences

口腔科　department of stomatology

口腔外科　oral surgery

口腔医院　oral hospital

口腔专业　specialty of stomatology

库存　inventory

库存(资金)周转次数　inventory

　turnover/turns

库存物资　material stocks

跨文化传播　cross-

　culture propagation

会计报表　accounting statement

会计账簿　account book

会计准则　accounting standard

扩展性　expansion

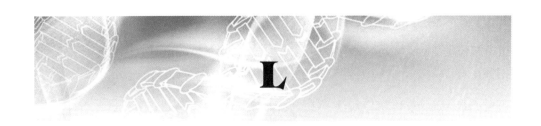

L

拉丁方设计 latin squares design

蓝盾 Blue Shield

蓝十字 Blue Cross

劳保医疗 labor health service

劳保医疗制度 labor insurance scheme

劳动安全 work safety

劳动保险 labour insurance

劳动和社会保障 labor and social security

劳动和社会保障部 Ministry of Labour and Social Security

劳动力 labor force

劳动平均产量 average product of labour

劳动生产率 productivity of labor

劳动用工制度 employment system

劳务费 labor cost

老年科 department of geriatrics

类似推理 analogize

类随机对照试验 quasi-randomized controlled trial

类推预测法 analogy method

of forecast

累积盈亏 accumulated profit or loss

累积折旧 accumulated depreciation

累计发病率 cumulative incidence rate

累计失败率 cumulative failure rate

累计死亡率 cumulative death rate

离散变量 discrete variable

离散度 discretion

离散型 discrete type

离散型分布 discrete distribution

离退休干部局 retiring cadre office

离退休人员基本养老金 basic pensions for retirees

离退休人员养老金 pensions to retired employees

理疗 physical therapy

理疗室 physiotherapy room

理疗医师（士） physiotherapist

理疗专业 specialty of physical therapy

理论解释 theoretical interpretation

理论模型 theoretical model

理论收益　theoretical profit

理事会　council

理想体重　ideal weight

理性　rationality

理性决策　rational decision making

理性预期　rational expectations

历史性对照研究　historical controlled trial

立法　legislation

立法解释　legislative interpretation

立法者　legislator

利润　profit

利润分配　profit distribution

利润函数　profit function

利润控制　profit control

利润率　profitability

利润水平　profits level

利润最大化　profit maximization

利他价值　altruistic value

利息率　interest rate

利息收入　interest revenue

利益冲突　conflict of interests

利益分布　distribution of benefits

利益相关者　stakeholder

利用　utilization

例外管理法　management by exception

例行检验　routine inspection

隶属关系　subjection rapport；relationship of administrative subordination

连抢救组　rescue group of company

连锁经营模式　chain-store operations

连锁医院　chain hospital

连卫生室　company medical room

连卫生员　medical corpsman

连续函数　continuous function

连续性变量　continuous variable

联合分析　conjoint analysis

联合国儿童基金会　United Nations Children's Emergency Fund（UNICEF）

联合国开发计划署　United Nations Development Programme（UNDP）

联合国人口基金会　United Nations Fund for Population Activities（UNFPA）

联合技术委员会　Joint Technical Committee

联合诊疗所　polyclinic

良性循环　beneficial cycle

量化测量　measure of quantity

量化考核　quantized appraisal

量化评价　quantitized assessment

疗养院　sanatorium

劣势治疗　dominated therapy

临床对照试验　controlled
clinical trial

临床服务满意度　satisfactory level
of clinical service

临床规章制度　clinical regulations

临床护理指挥　clinical
nursing conductor

临床技能　clinical skills
and competence

临床教授　clinical professor

临床结局　clinical outcome

临床经济学　clinical economics

临床决策分析　clinical
decision analysis

临床科室　clinical department

临床流行病学　clinical epidemiology

临床路径　clinical path（CP）

临床评价　clinical evaluation

临床审计　clinical audit

临床实践指南　clinical
practice guideline

临床试验　clinical trial

临床心理学　clinical psychology

临床信息系统　clinical
information system

临床研究申请　application for
clinical trial

临床研究证据　clinical
research evidence

临床药理基地　clinical
pharmacology base

临床药理学　clinical pharmacology

临床药效学
clinical pharmacodynamics

临床药学　clinical pharmacy

临床医疗质量　clinic medical quality

临床医师　clinician

临床证据　clinical evidence

临床证据手册　handbook of
clinical evidence

临床指南　clinical guideline

临界值　critical value

临时工　seasonal worker

遴选　select

灵敏度　sensitivity

零成本　zero cost

零弹性　zero elasticity

零基预算制度　a zero-base
budgeting system

零利润　zero economic profit

领导角色　leadership role

领导行为　leader behavior

领导艺术　art of leadership

领导者　leader

流动负债　current liabilities

流动人口　floating population

流动性　liquidity

流动资产　current assets

流行病　epidemic

流行病学　epidemiology

留治　holding for treatment

垄断　monopoly

垄断价格　monopoly price

垄断利润　monopoly profit

垄断行业　monopolized industry

垄断性竞争

　monopolistic competition

漏报　missing report

路径分析　path analysis

履行　comply

律师公证　lawyer notarization

率　rate

伦理　ethics

罗素指数　Rosser index

逻辑　logic

逻辑控制　logical control

逻辑斯谛回归　Logistic regression

逻辑斯谛回归模型　Logistic

　regression model

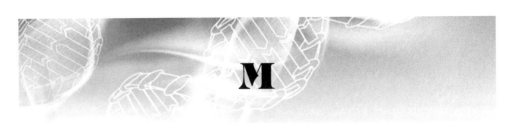

M

麻醉科　department of anesthesiology

麻醉师　anesthetist

马尔可夫模型　Markov model

买方垄断　monopsony power

卖方垄断　monopoly power

满意；满足　satisfaction

慢性呼吸疾病问卷　chronic respiratory disease questionnaire（RDQ）

慢性阻塞性肺疾病　chronic obstructive pulmonary disease（COPD）

盲法　blind method

盲态审核　blind review

没收　confiscate

每个医师的净收益　net revenue per physician

每年人口增加数　annual increment of the population

美国国家标准机构　American National Standard Institute

美国老人医疗保险处方药补偿计划　Medicare Prescription Drug Benefit

美国医疗机构评审联合委员会国际部医院评审标准　American Joint Commission International Accreditation Standards for Hospitals

美国医学院协会　American Association of Medical Colleges

美国质量控制学会　American Society for Quality Control

美国质量学会　American Society for Quality

门急诊人均费用　incoming fee per outpatient and emergency patient

门诊　outpatient service

门诊办公室　outpatient office

门诊部　department of out patient

门诊部主任　director of outpatient department

门诊服务　outpatient services

门诊管理　management of outpatient department

门诊护理　ambulatory nursing

门诊护理管理　ambulatory nursing management

门诊护士办公室　outpatient nurse's office

门诊患者　out patient

门诊患者人均医疗费用　average medical expense per outpatient

门诊人次数　outpatient visits

门诊申报　outpatient declaration

门诊质量指标　index of outpatient quality

门诊注射室　outpatient injection room

蒙特卡罗模拟　Monte Carlo Simulation

泌尿科　department of urology

泌尿科医师　urologist

免费医疗　free medical service

免税服务　tax-free service

免疫实验室　laboratory of immunology

面对面访问　face to face interview

描述性研究　descriptive study

灭菌　sterilization

民法　civil law

民防救护站　civil defense rescue station

民事　civilian; civil affairs

民事权利　civil right

民事诉讼　civil lawsuit

民事诉讼法　civil procedure law

民诉法院　court of common pleas

民营　private

民营化模式　privatization model

民营医院　private hospital

民主式领导　democratic leader

民族文化　national culture

敏感性分析　sensitivity analysis

命令　command

命令经济　command economy

模糊集　fuzzy set

模糊结构元　fuzzy structured element

模糊矩阵　fuzzy matrix

模糊聚类分析　fuzzy clustering analysis

模糊模型　fuzzy model

模糊数学　fuzzy mathematics

模糊统计　fuzzy statistic

模糊值函数　fuzzy-valued function

模糊综合评价　fuzzy comprehensive assessment

模拟编码　analog code

模拟测验　analogy test

模拟成本　simulated cost

模拟传输　analogue transmission

模拟法　analogue method

模拟计算　analog computation

模拟计算机　analogue computer

模拟技术　analogue technique

模拟控制　analog control

模拟量　analog quantity

模拟模型　analogue model

模拟数据　analog data

模拟数字转换　analogue

　digital conversion

模拟网络　analog network

模拟系统　analog system

模拟显示　analog display

模拟心理学　analog psychology

模拟信号　analog signal

模拟预测　simulating forecast

模式选择　model selection

模型参数　model parameter

摩擦成本　friction cost

母婴保健　maternal and infant care

　（MIC）

母婴同室　mother-infant rooming-in

目标　target；objective；goals

目标分解　target decomposition

目标管理　management by objectives

目标管理要素　target

　management elements

目标函数　objective function

目标激励　target stimulation

目标监测　target monitoring

目标结构　target structure

目标控制　target control

目标评价　goal-oriented evaluation

目标原则　target principle

目标展开　target expansion

目标战略学派　school of

　objective strategy

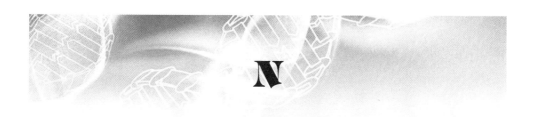

内部沟通　internal communication

内部环境　internal environment

内部活动　internal activity

内部评价　internal evaluation

内部审核；内部审计　internal audit

内部收益率　internal rate of return

内部因素　internal factor

内部治理结构　internal
governing structure

内部质量审核　internal
quality audits

内分泌科　department
of endocrinology

内分泌学　endocrinology

内涵　connotation

内剂量　internal dose

内镜室　endoscopy room

内科　department of
internal medicine

内科病房　medical ward

内科医师　doctor；physician

内科主任　director of the internal
medicine department

内控标准　internally
controlled standard

内容效度　content validity

内生变量　endogenous variable

内生性卫生资源　endogenous
health resources

内生性医疗资源　endogenous
medical resources

内省法　introspective method

内源性医院感染　endogenous
hospital infection

内源性资金　endogenous fund

内在动力　internal motive

内在矛盾　immanent contradiction

内在真实性　internal validity

纳什均衡　Nash equilibrium

耐药性　drug resistance；
drug tolerance

耐用品　durable goods

脑死亡　brain death

脑外科　department of
cerebral surgery

脑血管中心　cerebral vascular center

能力　competence

能力分析　ability analysis

能力管理　capacity management

拟合优度　goodness of fit

拟合优度检验　test of goodness

拟合优度指数　goodness of fit index

逆矩阵　inverse matrix

逆选择　adverse selection

年保险费　annual premium

年度计划　annual plan

年度考核　annual assessment

年净当量　annual net equivalent

年龄别死亡率　age-specific
　　death rate

年龄结构　age structure

年龄性别组成　age-sex composition

年龄组　age group

年增长率　annual growth rate

凝聚力　cohesion

纽带　vinculum

农村剩余劳动力　surplus
　　rural workers

农村剩余劳力的转移　the transfer of
　　rural surplus labors

农村税费改革　reform of rural taxes
　　and administrative charges

农业经济　agricultural economics

诺丁汉健康调查表　Nottingham
　　health profile

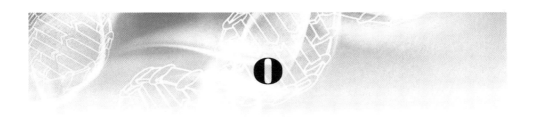

欧洲标准化委员会　European Committee for Standardization

欧洲五维生存质量量表　EuroQo l5-Dimensions（EQ-5D）

欧洲质量管理基金　European Foundation for Quality Management

欧洲质量奖　European Quality Award

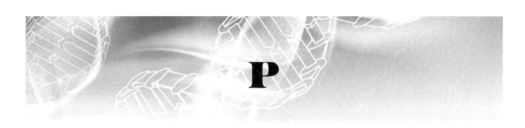

P

帕累托原理　Pareto principle

帕累托标准　Pareto criterion

帕累托改进　Pareto improvement

帕累托优化　Pareto optimality

排斥性;排他性　exclusion

排除标准　exclusion criteria

排队论　queuing theory

排队模型　queuing model

排队系统　queuing system

排列法　ranking method

排序稳定性分析方法　rank-order stability analysis（ROSA）

派生需求　derive demand

派生政策　derivative policy

判别分析　discriminant analysis

判定　judgement；assessment

判断抽样　judgmental sampling

判决　judgment

判例汇编　law report

培训　training

赔偿　compensation

赔偿限额　limitation of payments

赔付率　loss ratio

配对　matching

配对 t 检验　matched t-test

配对病例对照研究　matched case control study

配置　configuration

配置标准　distribution standard

配置程序　allocation procedure

配置室　collocation room

配置效率　allocation efficiency

配置指标　allocation index

批量采购　batch procurement

批量生产　batch production

批准　approval

批准阶段　approval stage

皮尔逊相关系数　Pearson correlation coefficient

皮肤科　department of dermatology

皮肤科医师　dermatologist

皮肤温度　skin temperature

皮肤学　dermatology

皮革马利翁效应　Pygmalion effect

匹配　match

偏差　deviation

偏度系数　coefficient of skewness

偏好　preference

偏回归系数　partial regression coefficient

偏离程度　deviation degree

偏倚　bias

频数分布　frequency distribution

频数分布表　frequency table

频数分布图　graph of frequency distribution

品牌　brand

品质提升　performance improvement（PI）

聘用制　engaging system

平等待遇　equal treatment

平衡表方法　balance-sheet approach

平均病床利用率　occupancy rate of beds；sickbed average usage rate

平均成本　average cost

平均成本定价法　average cost pricing

平均弹性系数　average elasticity

平均工资指数　index of average wage

平均固定成本　average fixed cost

平均剂量　average dose

平均减员　daily average casualties

平均开放病床数　average number of beds accessible

平均可变成本　average variable cost

平均利润　average profit

平均利润率　average rate of profit

平均每日出勤人数　average attendance per day

平均每日门诊人次数　average number of outpatients per day

平均年增长率　average annual growth rate

平均收益　average revenue

平均手术时间　mean operation time

平均数　average

平均税率　average tax rate

平均预期寿命　average life expectancy

平均值　medium value

平均住院日　average length of hospital stay

平均总成本　average total cost

平台　platform

平行比较法　paired comparison

平行效度　convergent validity

评定合格　assessment of conformity

评定量表法　rating scale method

评估　assessment

评估测量 evaluation and measurement

评估对象 auditing target

评价 evaluation

评价标准 evaluation standard

评价等级 evaluation grade

评价方法 evaluation method

评价工具 appraisal tool；evaluation tool

评价模型 evaluation model

评价型质量监督 quality supervision for approval

评价指标 evaluation index

评审 accreditation

评审程序 accreditation procedure

评审周期 accreditation period

普查 census

普通法 common law

普通人寿保险 ordinary life insurance

普外科 department of general surgery

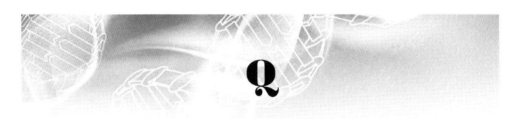

Q

期望 expectation

期望寿命 life expectancy

期望效用 expected utility

期望值 expected value

期望值原理 expected value principle

齐性检验 test for homogeneity

企业利益 enterprise interest

企业系统规划 business system planning

企业职工基本养老保险制度 the system of basic old age insurance for enterprise employees

企业资源计划 enterprise resources planning

启动 initiation

起付线（免赔额） deductible

起诉 indictment

起诉理由 cause of action

弃权 abstention

契约曲线 contract curve

器官移植 organ transplantation

前景 prospects

前景问题 foreground questions

前向设计 forward design

前沿 front edge

前沿兵站医院 combat zone hospital

前瞻性研究 prospective study

潜伏 incubation

潜伏期 incubation period

潜能 potential

潜意识 subconscious

潜在合作伙伴 potential partner

潜在减寿年数 potential years of life lost

强化理论 reinforcement theory

强势 strength

强制 compulsory；obligative

强制保险（义务保险） compulsory insurance

强制性 compulsory

强制性认证 compulsory certificate

抢救 rescue；salvage

抢救成功率 success rate in rescuing

抢救室 resuscitation room

侵入性操作 invasive manipulation

轻伤留治室 ward of holding lightly wounded

清洁区 cleanness section

情报会计 information accounting

请示 ask for instructions

穷人保险项目 medicaid program

区别定价 differentiated pricing

区间估计 interval estimation

区域 region

区域卫生规划 regional health planning

区域性救治 regional rescue

区组 block

区组随机化 block randomization

曲线拟合 curve fitting

趋势 tendency；trend

趋势外推法 trend extrapolation

趋同竞争 convergence competition

渠道 channel

全程灾备管理 whole course disaster management

全程质量管理 total quality management

全军保健领导小组办公室 Steering Office of Medical Department of CPLA

全科医师 general practitioner

全科医学 general medicine

全面成本管理系统 total cost management system

全面应用多种策略以开放阻塞性冠状动脉 Global Use of Strategies To open Occluded coronary arteries

全面质量管理 total quality management（TQM）

全面质量控制 total quality control（TQC）

权变理论 contingency theory

权力；权力机构 authority

权力结构 power structure

权利 right

权限 the limit of authority or power

权益调整 equity adjustments

权重 weight

缺乏弹性的 inelastic

缺乏效率 inefficiency

缺陷分析 flaw analysis

确定性模型 deterministic model

确定性治疗 definitive treatment

确认 validation

群体决策支持系统 group decision support system（GDSS）

群体免疫力 herd immunity

R

热原反应　pyrogen reaction

人才　talents

人工被动免疫　passive immunity

人工流产室　induced abortion room

人工系统　artificial system

人工智能　artificial intelligence（AI）

人工自动免疫　active immunity

人机对话　human-computer interaction

人际关系　human relation

人际交往能力　interpersonal skills

人际行为法　the interpersonal behavior approach

人均收入　income per capita

人均卫生费用　health expenditure per capita

人均药品费用　drug expenditure per capita

人口负增长　negative population growth（NPG）

人口更替水平　population replacement level

人口基数　population base

人口老龄化　aging of population

人口理论　population theory

人口零增长　zero population growth

人口流动　movement of population

人口年龄金字塔　population pyramid

人口年轻化　rejuvenation of population

人口普查　population census

人口统计　population statistics；demographics

人口研究　population studies

人口因素　demographic factor

人类发展指数　human development index

人力配置　manpower allocation

人力平衡　balance of manpower

人力投入　manpower input

人力资本　human capital

人力资本法　human capital approach

人力资源　human resources

人力资源管理　human resource management

人力资源规划　human resource planning

人力资源评估　evaluation of human resources

人力资源预测　prediction of human resources

人权　human rights

人权法案　civil right act

人群归因危险度　population attributable risk

人群归因危险度比　population attributable risk proportion

人群为基础的队列研究　population-based cohort study

人身保险　personal insurance

人身损害　personal injury

人时分析　person-time analysis

人事　staffing

人事档案管理　personnel archives management

人事管理　personnel management

人事司　department of personnel

人寿保险　life insurance

人为污染　anthropogenic

人性化服务　humanistic service

人员层次　personnel level

人员调配　personnel allocation

人员岗位培训　job training of personnel

人员结构　personnel structure

人员流动　turnover

人员培训　personnel training

人员数量　personnel quantity

人员素质　personnel quality

人员种类　personnel category

人员资格　qualification of personnel

认可　accreditation

认可标准　accrediting criteria

认可机构　accrediting body

认可实验室　accreditation of testing laboratories

认证方案　certification scheme

认证管理委员会　Certification Management Committee

认证活动　certification activity

认证机构　certification body

认证体系　certification system

认证体系成员　member of certification system

认证委员会　committee on certification

认证制度　the system of accreditation

认证质量工程师　certification

quality engineer

认证质量技术员 certification

quality technician

认证质量经理 certification

quality manager

认证质量审核员 certification

quality auditor

认知 cognition

认知方式 cognitive style

认知过程 cognitive process

认知技能 cognitive skill

认知结构 cognitive structure

认知失调 cognitive dissonance

认知心理学 cognitive psychology

任命制 system of appointing

任期考核 assessment of prefecture

任务准备 action/task preparation

妊娠 pregnancy

日本标准协会 Japanese

Standards Association

日常服务管理 daily

service management

日间医院 day care hospital

柔性 flexibility

柔性系统 flexible system

入院人数 number of admission

软科学 soft science

弱化 attenuation

弱势群体 disadvantaged groups

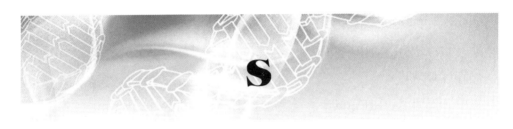

S

三防小组　NBC defense group

三级丙等医院　third-class hospital at grade 3

三级护理　three grade nursing

三级甲等医院　first-class hospital at grade 3

三级乙等医院　second-class hospital at grade 3

三级预防　tertiary prevention

三级质量控制　three-level quality control

三日确诊率　confirmed rate within three days

散点图　scatter plot

森林图　forest plots

筛选　screening

伤标　wound maker

伤病员分类　triage

伤部　location of injury

伤类　category of wounds

伤票　medical tag

伤情　wound condition

伤势　severity of wound

伤死　died of wounds

伤员　wounded

伤员流　wounded patient flow

伤员通过量　number of wounded passed

商品　commodity

商品化　commercialization

商品空间　commodity space

商品市场　commodity market

商品组合　commodity combination

商业保险　commercial insurance

商业价值　commercial value

商业伦理　business ethics

商业医疗保险　commercial medical insurance

上市后的监测　post marketing surveillance

上诉　appeal

上诉人　appellant

烧伤科　department of burn surgery

烧伤中心　burn center

设备　equipment

设备管理　equipment management

设备控制程序　equipment control procedure

设备年平均费用　annual average expense for equipment

设备完好率　equipment well-used rate

设备维修　equipment maintenance

社会保险　social insurance

社会保险机构　social security institution

社会保障　social security

社会保障体系　social security system

社会边际成本　marginal social cost

社会边际收益　marginal social benefit

社会成本　social cost

社会调查法　social investigation method

社会法人股　non-state-owned legal person's shares

社会服务　social service

社会福利　social welfare

社会福利金　social welfare fund

社会福利院　social welfare home

社会负担　social burdens

社会公共关系　social public relations

社会公共需要　common needs of the society

社会公益机构　social commonweal organization

社会共济　social joint relief

社会化　socialization

社会监督　society supervision

社会救助体系　social assistance system

社会统筹　overall social joint relief

社会统筹医疗基金　overall medical fund in all society

社会统筹与个人账户结合的模式 social unified raising and personal account system

社会卫生策略　social health strategy

社会稳定器　social stabilizer

社会相互影响　social interaction

社会效益　social benefit

社会心理学　social psychology

社会行为药学　social and behavioral pharmacy

社会需求调查法　the method of social need investigation

社会药学　social pharmacy

社会医疗保险　social medical insurance

社会医学　social medicine

社会责任　social responsibility

社会支持　social support

社会秩序　social order

社会资本　social capital

社交需要　social contact need

社交性赌博　social gambling

社交性饮酒　social drinking

社区　community

社区保健中心　community health care center

社区长期护理　community long-term nursing

社区筹资　community financing

社区服务　community service

社区护士　community nurse

社区康复服务　community-based rehabilitation

社区老年护理服务机构　community nursing home

社区卫生服务　community health service(CHS)

社区卫生服务机构　community health service institutions

社区卫生工作者　community health workers(CHW)

社区卫生教育　community health education(CHE)

社区卫生司　Community Sanitation Department

社区医疗　community medical care

社区医生　community practitioner

社区医学　community medicine

社区医院　community hospital

申报资料　claims data

申请　application；apply

申请人　applicant

申诉　complaint

身体力行　carry out by actual efforts

身心关系　psychosomatic relation

身心健康　physical and mental health

神经科专家　neurologist

神经内科　department of neurology

神经外科　department of neurosurgery

审查　review

审核；审计　audit

审核结论　audit conclusion

审核委托人　audit client

审核员　auditor

审批　examine and approve

肾内科　department of nephrology

肾移植　renal transplant（RT）

生产导向　production oriented

生产的最优条件　condition for efficiency in production

生产函数　production function

生产领域　production domain

生产率　productivity

生产能力　production capacity

生产效率　productive efficiency

生产要素　production factors

生产者均衡　producer equilibrium

生存分析　survival analysis

生存函数　survival function

生存检验　survival check

生存率　survival rate

生存年数　life years

生存曲线　survival curves

生存时间　survival time

生存质量效益法　quality of life benefit

生活标准　standard of living

生活补助　life subsidy

生活待遇　material amenities

生活方式　lifestyle

生活数量　quantity of life

生活质量指数　life quality index

生计问题　bread-and-butter issue

生理的需要　physiological needs

生理监控系统　physiological monitoring system

生命统计　vital statistics

生命指数　vital index

生命质量　quality of life

生命质量指数　quality of life index

生命周期　life cycle

生态比较研究　ecology comparison study

生态环境　ecological environment

生态建筑　ecological construction

生态流行病学　ecological epidemiology

生态趋势研究　ecology trend study

生态失衡　ecosystem disequilibrium

生态系统　ecosystem

生态研究　ecology study

生态医学模式　ecological medical model

生物半衰期　biological half-life

生物标志　biological marker

生物多样性　biodiversity

生物反馈　biofeedback

生物富集作用　bio-enrichment

生物统计学　biostatistics

生物-心理-社会医学模式　bio-psycho-social medical model

生物药学　biopharmacy

生物医学模式　biomedical model

生效　come into force

生育高峰　baby boom period

生殖保健　reproductive health

声誉　reputation

剩余控制权　residual rights
of control

剩余索取权　residual rights of claim

尸检　autopsy

失访　loss to follow-up；loss
to observation

失访偏倚　loss to follow-up bias

失能调整生命年　disability adjusted
life years

失效事件　failure event

失业保险　insurance for
the unemployed

失业保险金　unemployment
insurance benefits

失踪　missing

石膏室　plaster room

时间测量　measure of time

时间偏好　time preference

时间偏好率　rate of time preference

时间权衡法　time trade-off

时间损失成本　cost of lost time

时间效力　validity in time

时间效应偏倚　time effect bias

时间序列预测　time
series forecasting

时序　timing

实际利率　real interest rate

实际频数　actual frequency

实际需要　practical demand

实施　implementation

实施程序　implementation procedure

实施阶段　implement phase

实体　entity

实体关系模型　entity-
relationship model

实体系统　substantive system

实物形态　physical form

实物资本　material capital

实习　internship

实习医师　intern

实验对象　experiment object

实验对照　experiment control

实验法　experimental method

实验设计　experiment design

实验室　laboratory

实验室间的试验比较　inter-
laboratory test comparisons

实验室鉴定　laboratory qualification

实验室评定　laboratory assessment

实验室评定者　laboratory assessor

实验室认可报告　accredited laboratory test report

实验室认证　laboratory certification

实验室信息系统　laboratory information system

实验效率　efficiency of experiment

实验效应　experiment effect

实验研究　experiment study

实验研究设计　experiment study design

实验员　laboratory technician

食品及饮品许可证　food and drink permit

食品卫生　food hygiene； food sanitation

食品卫生法　food hygiene law

食品药品监督管理局　Food and Drug Administration（FDA）

食物添加剂　food additives

食物中毒　food poisoning

使命　mission

使用权　the right of use

使用效率　utilization efficiency

世界卫生组织　World Health Organization（WHO）

市场调查　market research

市场法规　market regulation

市场规模　market scale

市场机制　market mechanism

市场集中率　market concentration ratio

市场结构　market structure

市场经济　market economy

市场竞争　market competition

市场力　market power

市场前控制　premarket control

市场趋动型　market-driving type

市场失灵　market failure

市场细分　market segmentation

市场行为　market behavior

市场要素　market factor

市场营销　marketing

市场占有率　market share

市场政策　marketing policy

事故处理　settlement of accident； accident disposal

事件路径　event pathway

试点项目　pilot project

适度规模　moderate scale

适宜性　appropriateness

适宜性评价　appropriateness evaluation

适应性　suitability

适应性分组　adaptive randomization

适应需求　adapt to demand

适用范围　sphere of application

适用性　applicability

收费　charge

收容分类　reception triage

收入　income

收入补偿变量　compensating variation in income

收入弹性　income elasticity

收入等价变量　equivalent variation in income

收入分配制度　the system of income distribution

收益　revenue

收益递减　diminishing return

收益函数　revenue function

收益曲线　revenue curve

收益权　right to share; usufruct

收益最大化　revenue maximization

收支平衡　balance of revenue and expenditure

收支相抵点　break even point

手术　operation

手术安全　operation security

手术队　operation detachment

手术费　operation fee

手术后病死率　post-surgery mortality

手术率　operation rate

手术麻醉病死率　analgesia mortality

手术室　operation room

手术室管理　management of operation room

首因效应　primary effect

首诊　first encounter

寿命表　life table

寿命周期费用　life cycle cost

受试者工作特征曲线　receiver operator characteristic curve

受益人　beneficiary

兽医学　veterinary science

授权;委派　authorize; delegation

授予证书　grant certification

输出　output

输入　input

输液室　transfusion room

术后观察室　postoperative observation ward

术前准备室　preoperative preparation room

数据仓库　data warehouse

数据管理　data management

数据库　database

数据库管理系统　database management system

数据库系统　database system

数据挖掘　data mining

数据源定向的病历　source-oriented medical record

数据灾备　data backup

数学模型　mathematical model

数字减影血管造影技术　digital subtraction angiography

数字信号处理器　digital signal processor

双边协议　bilateral arrangement

双变量正态分布　bivariate normal distribution

双份录入　double entry

双盲法　double blind method

双盲试验　double blinded trial

双盲双模拟技术　double-blind and double-dummy technique

双模拟　double stimulation

双向　bilateral

双向性队列研究　ambispective cohort study

双向研究　ambidirectional study

双重分离　double dissociation

双重估计　double estimation

双重计算　double counting

双重权力结构　dual structure of authority

水平整合　horizontal integration

水灾控制法案　Flood Control Act

税收率　tax rate

司法法案　judicial act

司法机关　judicial organizations

司法鉴定　forensic appraisal

司法解释　judicial interpretation

司法文书　judicial documents

私人财产　private property

私人产品　private goods

私人成本　private cost

私人诊所　private clinic

私人资本　private capital

私营经济　private economy

思维　thinking

思维模式　thinking mode

死亡　decease；death；die

死亡率　mortality

死亡损失健康生命年　years of life lost

死因别死亡率　cause-specific death rate

四定　four administration points

四分位数间距　quartile range

四格表　fourfold table

似然比　likelihood ratio

似然比检验　likelihood ratio test

诉讼　litigation

诉讼法　procedure law

随访　follow-up

随访患病率研究　follow-up
prevalence study

随机变量　random variable

随机抽样　random sampling

随机对照试验　randomized
controlled trial

随机化　randomization

随机盲法对照临床试验　randomized
blind controlled clinical trial

随机模拟　random simulation

随机模型　stochastic model

随机平行对照试验　randomized

parallel control trial

随机区组设计　randomized
block design

随机双盲对照试验　stochastic double
blind controlled experiment

随机误差　random error

随机效应　random effect

随机效应模型　random effect model

随机应从设计　randomized
consent design

损伤　damage；harm；hazard；injury

缩减率　shrinkage

所得税费用　income tax expense

所有权　proprietary right

索赔的完全信度　full credibility for
claim numbers

索取权　claim right

T

胎心监护室　fetal monitor room

态度　attitude

滩头救护所　aid station on sea beach

弹性　elasticity

弹性法则　elasticity rule

探索性预测　exploratory forecasting

特点　characteristic

特定医疗费　special medical fee

特困行业和企业　industries and
enterprises in dire straits

特色管理
characteristic management

特色专科　featured discipline

特殊干预权　special right
to intervene

特许经营　government franchise

特异度　specificity

特诊科　department of
special treatment

特征值　eigenvalue

体制改革　system reform

体重指数　body mass index（BMI）

替代参数　substitution parameter

替代成本法　replacement cost

替代弹性　elasticity of substitution

替代品　substitutes

替代效应　substitution effect

替代要素　factor substitution

条件逻辑斯谛回归　conditional
logistic regression

条件反射　conditioned reflex（CR）

条件方差　conditional variance

条件评估　contingent evaluation
（CV）

条款　clause

贴现　discount

贴现率　discount rate

通货膨胀　inflation

通信　communication

通信管理
communication management

通用标准　general standard

通用量表　general instruments

通用药品　generic drugs

同等权利　equal right

同期效度　concurrent validity

同行评价 peer review

同行审查组织 peer review organization

同意 consent

同质性检验 tests for homogeneity

统筹管理 plan and manage as a whole

统筹规划 overall planning

统计 statistics

统计表 statistical table

统计调查 statistical survey

统计分析 statistical analysis

统计归纳 statistical induction

统计试验 statistical testing

统计图 statistical graph

统计效能（把握度） power

统计信息 statistical information

统计型决策 statistical decision

统计源期刊 journal of statistical source

统一化 unifying

头脑风暴 brain storming

投保人 policy holder or proposer

投标 bid；tender

投融资策略 financing

投入-产出 input-output

投入-产出模型 input-output model

投资 investment

投资成本 capital cost

投资公司 investment company

投资回报 return on investment

投资渠道多元化 diversification of investment

投资收益 investment income

投资损失 investment loss

透视室 fluoroscopy

透支 overdraft

突变论 mutation theory

突发事件 emergency events

图论 graph theory

图像存储与通信系统 picture archiving & communication system （PACS）

土地 land

土壤污染 soil contamination

团（旅）救护所 regiment or brigrade aid station

团队建设 team building

团队学习 team learning

团队智商 incorporation intelligence

团救护所 regimental aid station

团体人寿保险 group life insurance

团体愿景 group vision

退出 withdrawal

退休金;养老金　pension

退休基金　pension fund

托管模式　trusteeship model

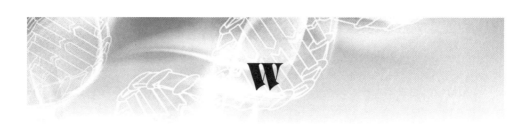

外部成本 external cost

外部环境 external environment

外部监督 external supervision

外部经济 external economy

外部收益;外部效益 external benefit

外部因素 external factor

外科 department of surgery

外科病房 surgical ward

外科护理学 surgical nursing

外科医师 surgeon

外科主任 director of the
surgical department

外来工 migrant worker

外来因素 extraneous factor

外生变量 exogenous variables

外推模型 extrapolation models

外延性 externality

外源性卫生资源 exogenous
health resources

外源性医疗资源 exogenous
medical resources

外源性医院感染 exogenous
hospital infection

完备性 completeness

完好率 the rate in good condition

完全成本 complete cost

完全寿命表 complete life table

完全随机化 complete randomization

完全随机设计 completely
random design

完全信息 complete information

完全正相关 perfect
positive correlation

完整性 integrity

玩忽职守 dereliction of duty

挽救后幸存年限 years of life saved

网络结构 network structure

网络图与网络计划 network chart
and network planning

网络系统管理 network
management system

往来账户 current account
with others

危机公关 crisis public relations

危险度 risk ratio

危险率 H probability of risk

危险行为　risk behavior

危险因素　risk factor

危重伤员观察室　holding-room for severely wounded

威胁　threat

微观调控　micro-control

微观核算型管理　intensive micro-management

微观决策　micro-decision

微生物　microbe

围生期　perinatal

围手术期　perioperative period

违法　contravene a law

唯学历论　academicalism

维护　maintenance

维修　maintain

伪造　forge；fabricate；forgery

委托-代理问题　principal-agent issues

委托权　power of attorney

委员会办公室　committee office

委员会草案　committee draft

卫勤保障　health service support

卫勤保障计划　plan of health service support

卫勤保障建议　proposal for health service support

卫勤保障预案　preliminary plan of health service support

卫勤部署　arrangement of health service

卫勤处　division of health service

卫勤分队　medical service unit

卫勤机动力量　mobilization of health service resources

卫勤机构配置　deployment of health service units

卫勤文书　health service documents

卫勤协同　coordination of health service institutions

卫勤训练　health service training

卫勤演习　health service maneuvers

卫勤医学研究室　department of health service research

卫勤预备力量　reserve of health service units

卫勤运力预计　estimation of health service transport

卫勤组织指挥　command and control of health service

卫生保健系统　consolidated health care systems

卫生保健资源　health care resources

卫生标准　hygienic standard；

sanitary standard

卫生部　Ministry of Public Health

卫生材料　medical materials

卫生材料费　the cost of
medical goods

卫生筹资　health financing

卫生处　medical division

卫生处长　chief of medical division

卫生床位资源　health bed resources

卫生法　health law

卫生法规　health regulation

卫生法制与监督司　Department of
Health Regulation and Supervision

卫生防疫　epidemic prevention

卫生防疫处　sanitary and anti-
epidemic division

卫生防疫队　sanitary and anti-
epidemic detachment

卫生防疫费　the cost of
epidemic prevention

卫生防疫检验所　sanitary and anti-
epidemic laboratory team

卫生防疫局　sanitary and anti-
epidemic administrative division

卫生防疫所　sanitary and anti-
epidemic element

卫生防疫侦察　sanitary and anti-

epidemic reconnaissance

卫生防疫专业　specialty of
epidemic prevention

卫生费用　health cost

卫生服务　health service

卫生服务成本　health care cost

卫生服务改革　health
service reforms

卫生服务机构资格认证联合委员会
Joint Commission on Accreditation
of Healthcare Organization

卫生服务体系　health service system

卫生管理　health management

卫生管理人员培训中心　health
administrator training center

卫生规划　health planning

卫生技术　health technology

卫生技术评估　health
technology assessment

卫生监督　health supervision

卫生监督办公室　Sanitary
Supervision Office

卫生减员　casualties due to
non effectives

卫生经费资源　health fund resource

卫生经济学　health economics

卫生经济政策　medical

economic policy

卫生局　health bureau

卫生科　medical section

卫生科长　chief of medical section

卫生立法　health legislation

卫生连　medical company

卫生旅　medical brigade

卫生评价　health evaluation

卫生勤务　health service

卫生人力资源　health

　　human resources

卫生设备资源　health

　　equipment resources

卫生事业机构　health service agency

卫生所　medical post

卫生体制改革　health care

　　system reform

卫生统计年报　annual report of

　　medical statistics

卫生统计学　health statistics

卫生统计月报　monthly report of

　　medical statistics

卫生系统　health system

卫生系统的反应水平　the level of

　　responsiveness of health system

卫生信息系统　health

　　information system

卫生行政部门　health authority

卫生行政处罚　administrative

　　penalty in respect of health

卫生学　hygieology；hygiology

卫生营　medical battalion

卫生员训练队　training detachment

　　for medical corpsmen

卫生账户　health account

卫生政策　health policy

卫生支出　health expenditure

卫生专业人员　health professional

卫生咨询　health consultation

卫生资源　health resources

卫生资源配置　health

　　resources distribution

卫生总费用　health

　　global expenditure

卫生总费用可变成本　total

　　health expenditure

卫生总预算　global health budgets

　　（GHB）

未来值　future value

胃镜室　gastroscopy room

文化　culture

文化氛围　cultural atmosphere

文件档案管理

　　document management

文书档案 document

文献检索 literature retrieval

稳定性 stability

稳定性假设 constancy assumption

污染区 polluted section

污水处理 sewage treatment

污水处理设备 sewage treatment equipment

污水排放量 sewage discharge

无残疾期望寿命 life expectancy free of disability

无差别 indifferent

无差异曲线 indifference curve

无偿调拨 appropriation

无偿使用 free use

无风险套利 arbitrage

无菌技术 aseptic technique

无菌区 asepsis section

无线通信 wireless communication

无限总体 infinite population

无效干预 invalid intervention

无效假设 null hypothesis

无形成本 invisible cost

无形资本 intangible capital

无形资产 immaterial assets；nonphysical assets

无序 disorder

无序竞争 disordered competition

无应答偏倚 non-response bias

物力 material resources

物有所值 value of money

物质的需要 material needs

物资储备量 material storage

物资的采购 material procurement

物资分类 material classification

物资库 material storehouse

物资平衡表 material balanced table

物资需要量 material requirement

误差 error

误差逆向传播模型 back propagation net-work

误工记录 record of labor-hours lost

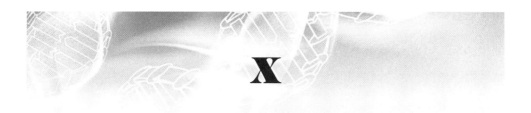

X

现场控制　field control

现场试验　field trial

现代管理制度　contemporary
　　management system

现代经营管理　modern
　　operational management

现代人力资源管理　modern human
　　resources management

现代医学模式　modern
　　medical model

现代医院　modern hospital

现代医院护理管理　modern
　　nursing management

现金分析　cash analysis

现金流量　cash flow

现况分析　situational analysis

现时寿命表　current life table

现收现付　pay as you go

现值　present value

线图　line graph

线性规划　linear programming

线性规划数学模型　linear
　　programming mathematical model

线性需求函数　linear
　　demand function

献血　blood donation

乡镇企业　township enterprises

相对价格　relative price

相对危险度　relative risk

相关法律问题　relative
　　legal problem

相关分析法　correlative
　　analysis method

相关矩阵　correlation matrix

相关系数　correlation coefficient

相关性分析　correlation analysis

相关因素预测　relative factor
　　forecasting method

相关指数　correlation index

相互影响　influence each other

相互制约　mutual control

相似接近度　similar approach degree

相似模拟　analog simulation

箱式图　box plot

向心力　centripetal force

项目　item

项目经理　program manager

项目评估和研究技术　program
　　evaluation research technology

项目实际投入额　factual input to
　　the project

削价　price cut

消毒　disinfection

消毒隔离　disinfection isolation

消毒供应室　sterilization and medical supply room

消毒供应中心　sterile supply centre

消毒管理　management of antisepsis

消费　consumption

消费可能　consumption possibility

消费空间　consumption space

消费心理学　consumer psychology

消费者　consumer

消费者均衡　consumer equilibrium

消费者理论　consumer theory

消费者偏好　consumer preference

消费者剩余　consumer surplus

消费者行为　consumer behavior

消费者选择　consumer choice

消费者优化　consumer optimization

消费者预算线　consumer's budget line

消费组合　consumption combination

消化科　department of gastroenterology

销毁　destroy；ruin

销货成本　cost of goods sold

销货收入　sales revenue

销售价格　sales price

销售利润　sales profit

销售量　sales volume

效果　effectiveness

效率　efficiency

效率参数　efficiency parameter

效率工资　efficiency wage

效能　efficacy

效益　benefit

效益-成本比率　benefit-cost ratio

效益分析　benefit analysis

效益原则　benefit principle

效应标志　biomarker of effect

效应尺度　effect magnitude

效应量　effect size

效用　utility

效用函数　utility function

效用理论　utility theory

效用最大化　utility maximization

校正　correction

协变量　covariate

协调　coordination

协调发展　coordinated development

协调系统　coherent system

协调性　concordant

协方差分析　analysis of covariance

协商　negotiation

协同效应　synergy effect

携带者　carrier

心导管室　DSA room

心电图室 electrocardiogram room

心功能室 heart function
　　examination room

心理过程 mental process

心理活动 mental activity

心理技术学 psychotechnics

心理健康 mental health

心理能动性 mental activism

心理素质 psychological quality

心理维度 psychological dimension

心理物理学 psychophysics

心理物理学方法
　　psychophysical method

心理现象 mental phenomenon

心理学 psychology

心理应激 psychological stress

心理运动 psychomotor

心向量室 vector-cardiography room

心血管病医师 cardiologist

心音图室 phono-cardiography room

心脏病科 department of cardiology

心脏外科 department of
　　cardiac surgery

心智模式 mental mode

新观念 new idea

新生儿 neonate

新生儿重症监护室 neonate

intensive care unit

新特药房 new and special drugstore

新闻媒介 news media

新兴产业 newly rising industry

新药申请 new drug application

新药审批 new drug approval

新职工上岗前培训 pre-education
　　and training for new
　　staff members

薪酬 reward

薪资支出 payroll expense

信度 reliability

信度因子 credibility factor

信访 postal interview

信息 information

信息编码 information encoding

信息不对称 asymmetric information

信息成本 information cost

信息储存 information storage

信息处理 information handling

信息处理系统 information
　　processing system

信息传递 information transmission

信息对称 symmetry of information

信息反馈 information feedback

信息方法 information method

信息访问 information access

信息非对称性

　　information asymmetry

信息分布　information distribution

信息服务　information service

信息革命　information revolution

信息管理　information management

信息规划　information planning

信息化管理

　　informatization management

信息化社会　information society

信息获取　information acquisition

信息技术　information technology

信息加工　information processing

信息价值的分析　value of

　　information analysis

信息检索　information retrieval

信息接收者　information receiver

信息经济　information economics

信息科学　information science

信息量　information quantity

信息流　information flow

信息论　information theory

信息偏倚　information bias

信息收集　information collection

信息输出　information output

信息体系结构　information

　　system architecture

信息系统　information system

信息载体　information carrier

信息政策与法规　information policy

　　and law

信息主管　chief information officer

信息转换　information conversion

信息资源　information source

信息资源管理　information

　　resources management

信息组织　information organization

信用　credit

信用保险　credit insurance

信誉　credit and reputation

兴奋剂　stimulants

星级护理　star-nursing

刑法　criminal law

刑事诉讼法　criminal procedure law

刑事责任　criminal responsibility

行为尺度评定量表　behaviorally

　　anchored rating scales（BARS）

行为方式　behavior style

行为科学　behavioral science

行为修正　action emending

行为药学　behavioral pharmacy

行业垄断　monopolized industry

行政处分　administrative punishment

行政法　administrative law

行政干预

　　administrative intervention

行政纲领;法定纲要

　　official compendium

行政管理　administrative

　　management（ADM）

行政机关的裁决　agency stage

行政强制执行

　　administrative enforcement

行政人员　administrative staff

行政手段　administrative method

行政职务　administrative duty

行政指令　administrative command

形式多样化　diversification of forms

型式批准　type approval

型式评价　type evaluation

性别比率　sex ratio

性病科　department of venereology

性质　characteristics

胸外科　department of

　　thoracic surgery

胸外科医师　cardiac surgeon

休假　vacation

休养所　rest home

修订　amendment

修缮费　repair and maintenance cost

修正均数　adjusted means

修正因子　correction factor

虚拟企业　virtual organization

需求　demand

需求变化　change in demand

需求表　demand schedule

需求弹性　demand elasticity

需求的交叉弹性　cross elasticity

　　of demand

需求定理　law of demand

需求分析　demand analysis

需求管理　demand management

需求函数　demand function

需求价格　demand price

需求价格弹性　price elasticity

　　of demand

需求量　quantity of demand

需求量变化　change in

　　quantity demanded

需求评估　need assessment

需求曲线　demand curve

需求收入弹性　income elasticity

　　of demand

需求向下倾斜规律　law of

　　downward-sloping demand

需求要素　factor demand

需求周期　demand cycle

需要　need

需要评估　need analysis

许可证　license

序贯决策　sequential decision

序贯设计　sequential design

序贯试验　sequential trial

叙述法　narrative method

续保　renew

续约　renewal of contract

选择性偏倚　selection bias

学科　discipline

学科技术资源　discipline technology resources

学科建设　subject construction；discipline construction

学科资源　discipline resources

学习型社会　learning society

学习型医院　learning hospital

学习型组织　learning organization

学习制度　learning system

血库　blood bank

血透室　hemodialysis room

血液安全　blood security

血液科　department of hematology

血液实验室　blood laboratory

血液透析　hemodialysis（HD）

血液透析机　hemodialysis machine

血液制品　blood product

血源传播性疾病　bloodborne disease

寻租　rent seeking

巡诊　round

循环质量控制　circle quality control

循证儿科学　evidence-based pediatrics

循证妇产科学　evidence-based gynecology & obstetrics

循证护理　evidence-based nursing

循证决策　evidence-based decision-making

循证内科学　evidence-based internal medicine

循证筛选　evidence-based selection

循证外科学　evidence-based surgery

循证卫生保健　evidence-based health care

循证医学　evidence-based medicine

循证医学标准　evidence-based medical standard

循证医学教育　evidence-based medical education

循证医学资源　evidence-based medical resources

循证诊断　evidence-based diagnosis

训练费　training expense

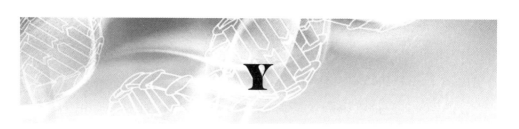

Y

压力　pressure

牙科　department of dentistry

牙科学　dentistry

牙科医师　dentist

哑变量　dummy variables

亚队列研究　sub-cohort study

亚临床感染;无症状性感染
　　subclinical infection

亚洲标准咨询委员会　Asian
　　Standard Advisory Committee

亚组分析　subgroup analysis

延期变动成本　deferred variable cost

延误诊疗　delay to diagnose
　　and treat

严格评价　critical appraisal

言语治疗师(士)　speech therapist

研发　research & development

研究论文　research papers

研究所　research institute

眼科　department of ophthalmology

眼科学　ophthalmology

眼科医师　oculist

眼科专家　ophthalmologist

演绎法　deduction

验后比　post-test odds

验后概率　post-test probability

验前比　pre-test odds

验前概率　pre-test probability

验收检验　acceptance inspection

验证　verification

验证性研究　confirmatory study

阳性预测值　positive
　　predictive value

养老保险　endowment insurance

养老保障制度　the retirement
　　pension system

样本　sample

药材保管　storage of
　　medical supplies

药材报废　scrapping of
　　medical supplies

药材报废标准　scrapping criteria of
　　medical supplies

药材补给标准　standard of
　　medical supply

药材仓库　depot of

medical materials

药材储备 reserve of
medical supplies

药材储备定额 quota reserve of
medical supplies

药材处 division of medical supplies

药材防护 protection of
medical supplies

药材分配 distribution of
medical supplies

药材供应 medical supply

药材供应标准 medical
supply standard

药材供应体制 system of
medical supply

药材购买 procurement of
medical supplies

药材核算 medical supply accounting

药材库存量 stock amount of
medical supplies

药材库房 store-house for
medical supplies

药材流动储备 mobile reserve of
medical supplies

药材轮换更新 rotating renewal of
medical supplies

药材日常储备 routine reserve of

medical supplies

药材统计 medical supply statistics

药材消耗限额 consumption quota of
medical supplies

药材预算 estimation of requirement
of medical supplies

药材战略储备 strategic reserve of
medical supplies

药材战术储备 tactical reserve of
medical supplies

药材战役储备 campaign reserve of
medical supplies

药房 pharmacy

药房管理 pharmacy management

药剂科 section of
pharmaceutical preparation

药剂人员 paramedics

药局主任 chief of pharmacy

药库 pharmacy store

药库主任 director of
pharmacy store

药理科 department
of pharmacology

药品 drug

药品安全 drug safety

药品不良反应监测 adverse drug
reactions monitoring

药品采购　procurement of drugs

药品参考定价　reference pricing
　of drugs

药品定价　prices for medicines

药品定价管制　pricing control
　of drugs

药品管理办法　drug
　management method

药品管理法　pharmaceutical
　management law

药品价格　drug price

药品监督员　drug inspector

药品经营　drug operation

药品经营许可证　license for
　pharmaceutical trading

药品开发　pharmaceutical research
　and development

药品零售　retail of drugs

药品批号　drug batch number

药品器材局　Medicine and
　Supplies Division

药品生产质量管理规范　good
　manufacturing practice for drugs
　（GMP）

药品市场失灵　dysfunction of
　pharmaceutical market

药品销售部门　department of

drug selling

药品营销与管理　pharmaceutical
　marketing and management

药品招标　pharmaceutical bidding

药品支出　drug expenditure

药品质量标准　drug quality standard

药品质量管理　drug
　quality management

药品质量监督　drug quality control

药师　pharmacist

药师资格考试制度　examination
　system for
　pharmacists' qualification

药士；助理药师　assistant pharmacist

药事管理
　pharmaceutical administration

药事管理委员会　pharmaceutical
　administration committee

药事管理学
　pharmacy administration

药物保险计划　Pharmaceutical
　Benefits Scheme（PBS）

药物不良反应　adverse drug reaction

药物非临床研究质量管理　good
　laboratory practice（GLP）

药物分析　drug analysis

药物和治疗委员会　pharmacy and

therapeutics committee

药物化学　medicinal chemisty

药物经济学　pharmacoeconomics

药物经济学分析

　　pharmacoeconomics analysis

药物利用　drug utilization

药物利用度评估　drug use evaluation

药物利用指数　drug utilization index

药物临床试验管理规范　good clinical

　　practice（GCP）

药物流行病

　　学　pharmacoepidemiology

药物效果　effect of medicine

药物效用　utility of drugs

药物治疗　medication treatment

药物治疗的社会经济评价

　　socioeconomic evaluation of

　　drug therapy

药学保健　pharmaceutical care

药学部　department of pharmacy

药学服务　pharmacy service

药学教研室　teaching and research

　　section of pharmacy

药学教育　pharmaceutical education

药学实践　pharmacy practice

药学事业

　　pharmaceutical undertaking

药政管理　drug administration

要求　want

野战　field

野战病历　field medical history

野战传染病医院　field hospital for

　　infectious diseases

野战毒剂伤医院　field hospital for

　　war gas-injury

野战内科学　war internal medicine

野战轻伤病医院　field hospital for

　　lightly wounded

野战手术室　field operation room

野战输血　field blood transfusion

野战外科学　war surgery

野战医疗队　field medical team

野战医疗所　field aid station

野战医院　field hospital

业绩　performance

业绩考评　achievement evaluation

业绩评定表　rating scales method

业绩评价　performance measurement

业务成本　operational costs

业务副院长　vice dean in charge of

　　medical services

业务收入　agency revenue

业务拓展　business development

业务专长　specialized skill

一级丙等医院　third-class hospital at grade 1

一级甲等医院　first-class hospital at grade 1

一级乙等医院　second-class hospital at grade 1

一级预防　primary prevention

一线医院　first line hospital

一氧化碳中毒　carbon monoxide poisoning

一致　consensus

一致性　consistency

一致性效度　agreement validity

医护质量　medical care quality

医患关系　doctor-patient relationship

医教部　medical and teaching administration

医疗安全　medical safety

医疗安全防范　medical safety precaution

医疗安全管理　medical safety management

医疗保健　medical health care

医疗保健协会　healthcare associations

医疗保险　medical insurance

医疗保险法　medical insurance law

医疗保险范围　package of medical insurance

医疗保险费　medical insurance premium

医疗保险管理　medical insurance management

医疗保险管理信息系统　medical Insurance management information system（MIMIS）

医疗保险机构　medical insurance institution

医疗保险基金　funds of medical insurance

医疗保险监督　supervision of medical insurance

医疗保险卡　medical insurance overage card

医疗保险学　medical insurance science

医疗保险政策　hospitalization insurance policy

医疗保险政策分析　hospitalization insurance policy analysis

医疗保险制度　medical insurance system

医疗保险制度改革　reform of

medical insurance system

医疗保障组　medical support group

医疗差错　medical error

医疗成本　medical cost

医疗成本管理　medical
cost management

医疗成本核算　medical
cost accounting

医疗成本控制　medical cost control

医疗处　division of
medical treatment

医疗队　medical detachment

医疗废物　medical waste

医疗废物管理　the management of
medical waste

医疗费　medical expense

医疗费用　medical expenditure

医疗费用补偿　compensation of
medical cost

医疗风险　medical risk

医疗风险管理　medical
risk management

医疗服务　health service

医疗服务价格　the price of
medical service

医疗服务量　volume of medical care

医疗服务市场　medical

service market

医疗服务提供方　health
care provider

医疗服务提供体系　healthcare
delivery system

医疗服务质量　medical
service quality

医疗改革　health care reform

医疗管理　medical administration

医疗管理基本原则　fundamental
principles of medical management

医疗管理局　Medical Treatment
Administrative Division

医疗规章制度　rule and regime of
medical care

医疗合作制度　medical
cooperation system

医疗后送　medical evacuation

医疗后送体制　medical
evacuation system

医疗后送文件袋　documents for
medical evacuation

医疗护理中心　medical &
nursing center

医疗活动　medical activities

医疗机构　medical institutions

医疗集团　medical services group

医疗技术标准　medical technique standard

医疗技术标准体系　medico technical standard system

医疗技术操作标准　medico technical operation standard

医疗技术方法标准　medico technical method standard

医疗技术风险　the risk of medical technology

医疗教育和培训　medical education and training

医疗纠纷　medical dispute

医疗决策　medical decision making

医疗决策制定协会　Society for Medical Decision Making

医疗科室　departments of medical care

医疗评价　medical evaluation

医疗器械　medical devices

医疗器械检修所　medical instrument repairing shop

医疗侵权诉讼　medical right infringement lawsuit

医疗设备　medical equipments

医疗设备代码　code of medical equipment

医疗实践　medical practice

医疗市场　medical service market

医疗市场分析　medical market analysis

医疗市场环境　medical market environment

医疗事故　medical malpractice

医疗事故发生率　incidence of malpractice

医疗事故技术鉴定　technical appraisals of malpractice

医疗事故鉴定　medical accident appraisal

医疗收入　income from medical services

医疗收益　gain from medical treatment

医疗损失比例　medical loss ratio

医疗体系　medical system

医疗体制改革　the reform of medical system

医疗卫生行政管理　healthcare administration

医疗文书　medical document

医疗系统反应性　the responsiveness of health system

医疗系统构件　elements of

medical system

医疗系统总体反应性 total responsiveness of health system

医疗系统组成 form of medical system

医疗项目成本核算 item-based cost accounting

医疗效果 medical effect

医疗信息与管理系统协会 Healthcare Information and Management Systems Society（HIMSS）

医疗需求 medical demand

医疗责任 medical obligation

医疗责任风险 the risk of medical obligation

医疗制度 medical care system

医疗制度改革 medicare system reform

医疗质量 medical quality

医疗质量标准 medical quality standard

医疗质量改进法 health care quality improvement

医疗质量管理 medical quality management

医疗质量控制 medical

quality control

医疗质量控制标准 control standard of medical quality

医疗质量控制点 control point of medical quality

医疗质量控制系统 control system of medical quality

医疗质量评价体系 medical quality evaluation system

医疗质量评价指标 index on medical treatment quality

医疗质量评鉴 audit quality of care

医疗质量要素 elements of medical quality

医疗秩序 medical order

医疗中心 medical center

医疗资源 medical resources

医疗资源结构 medical resource structure

医疗资源配置 medical resources allocation

医疗资源优化配置 optimum allocation of medical resource

医师办公室 doctor's office

医师的可获得性 physician availability

医师工作间 doctor's workshop

医师行医管理 physician practice management

医师诊断证明书 aeger

医师职业风险 the risk of medical practice

医师资格考试制度 examination system for doctors' qualification

医士 assistant doctor

医务部（处） medical administration division

医务部主任 chief of medical branch

医务人员 medical personnel；medical staff

医务人员认证 accreditation of medical staff

医学 medicine

医学参考值范围 medical reference range

医学技术 medical technology

医学技术人员 medical professionals

医学技术资源 medical technology resources

医学科技进步 medical science and technology progress

医学科学技术 medical science and technology

医学科学技术委员会 Council of Medical Sciences and Technology

医学伦理学 medical ethics

医学美容中心 medical cosmetic center

医学模式 medical model

医学情报 medical information

医学社会学 medical sociology

医学统计学 medical statistics

医学心理学 medical psychology

医学信息学 medical informatics

医学信息学欧洲联盟 European Federation for Medical Informatics

医学影像中心 medical image center

医学专科中心 specialized medical centre

医药市场机制 mechanism of pharmaceutical market

医药知识产权 medicine intellectual property rights

医用直线加速器 medical linear accelerator

医源性疾病 iatrogenic diseases

医院 hospital

医院安全文化 hospital culture of safety

医院本质文化 hospital nature culture

医院标准　hospital standard

医院标准化管理　hospital
management standardization

医院标准体系　hospital
standard system

医院财务预算　hospital
financial budgeting

医院财务状况　financial situation
of hospital

医院产出指标　hospital output index

医院成本管理　hospital
cost management

医院成本控制　hospital cost control

医院道德　hospital morals

医院发展　hospital development

医院发展战略　hospital
development strategy

医院费用控制　control of
medical cost

医院分级管理　hospital
stratified management

医院分级管理和评审　hierarchical
management and accreditation
of hospital

医院风尚　hospital fashion

医院福利费　hospital benefits

医院副院长　deputy director

of hospital

医院感染　hospital infection

医院感染管理　hospital
infection management

医院感染监测　hospital
infection monitoring

医院感染控制　hospital
infection control

医院感染流行病学　epidemiology in
hospital infection

医院工作效益指标　benefit index of
hospital work

医院功能分区　hospital
functional block

医院供应和分配系统　hospital supply
and distribution system

医院固定资产　hospital fixed assets

医院管理　hospital management

医院管理标准　hospital
management standard

医院管理部门　hospital
administrative department

医院管理架构　hospital
management structure

医院管理系统　hospital
management system

医院管理信息系统　hospital

management information system

医院管理学会　Hospital
Management Association

医院规模　hospital scale

医院宏观调控　hospital macroscopic
control and adjustment

医院后勤保障　hospital
logistics assurance

医院后勤服务产业化
industrialization of hospital
logistics service

医院后勤服务集约化　intensive
management of hospital
logistics service

医院后勤服务目标管理责任制
system of job responsibility in
management by objectives

医院后勤服务社会化　socialization
of hospital logistics service

医院后勤管理　hospital
logistic management

医院后勤管理体制　hospital logistics
management system

医院后勤现代化　modernization of
hospital logistics

医院护理管理　hospital
nursing management

医院环境　hospital environment

医院环境与卫生学管理　hospital
environment and
hygiene management

医院会计制度　hospital
accounting system

医院基础条件标准　basic
requirements of hospital settings

医院基金管理　hospital
fund management

医院绩效测量工具　hospital
performance measurement tools

医院绩效管理　hospital
performance management

医院绩效管理评价　hospital
performance
management evaluation

医院绩效管理体系　hospital
performance management system

医院绩效评估　function of hospital
performance assessment

医院绩效评估体系　hospital
performance assessment system

医院集团　group hospital

医院计算机信息系统　hospital
computerized information system

医院技术管理　hospital

technical management

医院价格指数　hospital price index

医院建筑　hospital architecture

医院建筑标准　architecture standard for hospital

医院建筑管理　hospital building management

医院建筑设备系统　hospital building equipment system

医院建筑组合形式　hospital building combination

医院交通运输系统　hospital traffic system

医院结构　hospital structure

医院经济管理　hospital economics management

医院经济核算　hospital economic accounting

医院经营管理　hospital operation management

医院经营管理战略　hospital management strategy

医院经营合作　hospital operation cooperation

医院经营决策　hospital operational decision

医院精神文化　hospital

spiritual culture

医院扩展系统　hospital expansion system

医院扩张　hospital expansion

医院领导　hospital leadership

医院领导体制　hospital leadership system

医院内部环境　hospital internal environment

医院内部审计　internal hospital audit

医院内感染　nosocomial infection；hospital infection

医院内环境管理　hospital internal environment management

医院排水制度　hospital drainage system

医院评价标准　hospital evaluation standard

医院评审委员会　commission on the accreditation for hospital

医院期望　hospital expectation

医院人本文化　human-oriented hospital culture

医院人力资源管理　hospital human resources management

医院人员编制　hospital

personnel organization

医院人员构成比 constituent ratio of all kind of staffs in hospital

医院设备 hospital equipment

医院设备分类 hospital equipment classification

医院设计和建设 hospital design and construction

医院设施 hospital facilities

医院审计 hospital auditing

医院生存危机 survival crisis of hospital

医院所有权 hospital proprietary right

医院特性 hospital characteristics

医院通信系统 hospital communication system

医院统计 hospital statistics

医院统计指标 hospital statistical index

医院图书馆 hospital library

医院外部环境 hospital external environment

医院外环境管理 hospital external environment management

医院卫生技术人员构成比 constituent ratio of all kinds of

health and technical staff in hospital

医院卫生学管理 hospital hygienic management

医院文化 hospital culture

医院文化冲突 hospital culture shock

医院文化的道德建设 moral construction in the hospital culture

医院文化的核心 the core of hospital culture

医院文化的角色 the role of hospital culture

医院文化的衰败 disruption of hospital culture

医院文化共同体 hospital cultural community

医院文化构建 construction of hospital culture

医院文化观念 hospital culture conception

医院文化规模 hospital culture scale

医院文化机制 mechanism of hospital culture

医院文化评测 measurement of hospital culture

医院文化实践 practice of hospital culture

医院文化特性　character of
hospital culture

医院文化网络　hospital
culture network

医院文化影响　the influence of
hospital culture

医院文化转化　transformation of
hospital culture

医院污水　hospital sewage

医院污水处理　hospital waste-
water disposal

医院物质文化　hospital
matter culture

医院物资定额管理　hospital material
quota management

医院物资管理　hospital
material management

医院系统工程　hospital
system engineering

医院消防系统　hospital
firefighting system

医院信息　hospital information

医院信息管理　hospital
information management

医院信息系统　hospital
information system

医院行为文化　hospital

behavior culture

医院行政管理　hospital
administrative management

医院药局　pharmacy of hospital

医院用药目录　formulary

医院院长　director of hospital

医院运行系统　hospital
operation system

医院噪声　hospital noise

医院债权　hospital creditor's rights

医院战备　hospital war preparation

医院战略　hospital strategy

医院战略管理　hospital
strategy management

医院战略重点　hospital
strategy priority

医院哲学　hospital philosophy

医院支持系统　hospital
support system

医院职能机构　hospital
functional structure

医院质量　hospital quality

医院质量标准化　hospital
quality standardization

医院质量管理　hospital
quality control

医院质量管理体系　hospital quality

management systems

医院质量满意度　hospital quality satisfaction

医院资本　hospital capital

医院资本运营　hospital capital management

医院资产　hospital asset

医院资产重组　hospital capital recomposition

医院宗旨　hospital tenet

医院综合效益评价　hospital comprehensive benefits evaluation

医院总成本核算　total cost accounting of a hospital

医政分离　separate medicine and authority

医政合一　integration medicine with authority

医政司　department of medical administration

医政司长　director of medical department

医嘱　advice for the patient；doctor's orders

依从性　compliance

依法管理　law-based management

仪器　instrument

仪器室　instrument room

遗传　inheritance

遗传流行病学　genetic epidemiology

遗传学　genetics

疑难病例　intractable case

以患者为中心　patient-centred

以人为本　human-oriented

以资源为基础的相对价值标准　resource based relative value system（RBRVs）

义务　liability；obligation

异质产品　heterogeneous product

异质性检验　tests for heterogeneity

译码　decode

易感人群　susceptible population

易感性　susceptibility

易感性生物标志　biomarker of susceptibility

疫苗　vaccine

疫情　epidemic situation

疫情报告系统　infectious disease report system

疫情管理　management of epidemic situation

疫情监测　epidemic situation monitoring

意识　consciousness

意愿接受法 willingness to accept（WTA）

意愿支付法 willingness to pay（WTP）

因果联系 cause-effect relationship

因食物而引起的感染与中毒 food-borne infection and intoxication

因食物而引起的疾病 food-borne disease

因素评价法 factor evaluation

因子分析 factor analysis

阴性预测值 negative predictive value

银行借款 bank loan

引用偏倚 citation bias

隐私权 the right of privacy

隐性成本 implicit cost

隐性感染 latent infection

隐性效益 intangible benefit

应变策略 contingency strategy

应变量 dependent variable

应变准则 contingency rule；strain criteria

应付账款 accounts payable

应急管理 emergency-response management

应急机动医院 emergency mobile hospital

英国工程标准协会 British engineering standards associations

婴儿死亡率 infant mortality rate

盈余 surplus

营救护所 battalion aid station

营利性医院 profitable hospital

营利性组织 for-profit organization

营卫生所 battalion medical post

营销策略 marketing strategy

营养不良 malnutrition

营养师 nutritionist

营养与食品卫生学 nutrition and food hygiene

营业收入 operating revenue

营业外收入 non-operating revenue

硬件建设 hardware construction

硬件资源 hardware resources

用药频度 administration frequency

优化 optimization

优化配置 optimize allocation

优惠政策 preferential policy

优劣程度 fit and unfit level

优生优育 eugenics

优胜劣汰 survival of the fittest

优势 advantage

优势互补 complement each other

优势-机会战略 strength-opportunity strategy

优势-威胁战略 strength-threat strategy

优先者提供组织 preferred provider organization(PPO)

优质服务 high quality service

优质资产 high quality capital

幽门螺杆菌 Helicobacter pylori (Hp)

尤登指数 Youden's index

铀中毒 uranium poisoning

有偿转让 compensable transfer; remunerative transfer

有线通信 wire communication

有限总体 finite population

有限总体校正因子 finite population correction factor

有效表达 effective presentation

有效沟通 effective communication

有效管理 effective management

有效规模 efficient scale

有效配置 effective allocation

有形资产 tangible assets

有序 order

有序竞争 orderly competition

诱导需求 induced demand

语言偏倚 language bias

预测 prediction

预测程序 forecasting procedure

预测学 forecast science

预防 prevention

预防保健服务模式 preventive health service model

预防保健科 department of health care and prevention

预防保健体制 prevention and health care system

预防保健网络 prevention and health care network

预防措施 preventive measures

预防服务 prevention service

预防和控制 prevention and control

预防监督体制 prevention and supervision system

预防性风险 preventable risk

预防医学 preventive medicine

预付 prepayment

预付保险费 prepaid insurance

预付费用 prepaid expenses

预付退休金 prepaid pension cost

预付薪资 prepaid payroll

预付制度 prospective payment system

预付租金　prepaid rents

预后　prognosis

预后因素　prognostic factor

预后指数　prognostic index

预警机制　early-warning system

预期结果　planned results

预期目标　expected objective

预算　budget

预算赤字　budget deficit

预算管理　budget management

预算线　budget line

预算盈余　budget surplus

预算影响　budget impact

预算约束　limited budget

阈值分析　threshold analysis

原料药　drug substance

原始研究　primary studies

原始研究证据　primary
　research evidence

院长负责制　system of president
　in charge

院内分娩死亡率　delivery mortality
　in hospital

院内感染率　hospital infection rate

院内新生婴儿死亡率　infant
　mortality rate in hospital

约束　restraint

约束理论　theory of constraints
　（TOC）

约束力　constraint force

孕产妇死亡率　maternal
　mortality rate

运筹学　operational research

运动医学科　department of
　sport medicine

运输设备　transportation equipment

运行机制　operational mechanism

运行效率;运营效率
　operating efficiency

运营方式　operational style

运营系统　operational system

晕轮效应　dizzy wheel effect

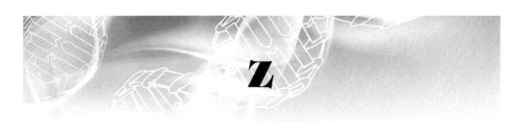

Z

灾备　disaster preparedness

灾备管理　disaster management

灾备训练　disaster preparedness training

灾害损失　casualty loss

灾害医学　disaster medicine

灾难备份　disaster backup

灾难恢复　disaster recovery

再保险公司　reinsurance company

暂付款　temporary payments

暂收款　temporary receipts

早期治疗　early treatment

噪声引起耳聋　noise-induced deafness

责任；职责　responsibility

责任感　consciousness of responsibility

责任心　responsibility

增量成本效果比　incremental cost effectiveness ratio

增量分析　incremental analysis

增量资本　increment capital

增量资产　increment asset

增强作用　synergism

债权人　creditor

占有率　occupancy rate

占有权　corporeal right

战备储备　combat readiness storage

战斗减员　battle casualties

战斗支援医院　combat support hospital

战俘医院　hospital for prisoners of war

战救 5 项技术　five techniques of first aid

战救药材　medical supplies for first aid in war

战救药材基数　basic unit of medical supplies for field first aid

战略　strategy

战略部署　strategy deployment

战略方针　strategic guideline

战略管理　strategy management

战略管理模型　strategy management model

战略规划　strategy planning

战略后方　strategic rear

战略决策　strategic decision

战略控制　strategy control

战略目标　strategic objective

战略实施　strategy implementation

战略实施体系　strategy
　implementation system

战略实施效果　strategy
　implementation effect

战略协作　strategic cooperation

战区基地医院　base hospital of
　the front

战伤减员　wounded in action

战时常备药材　standing medical
　supplies in wartime

战术　tactics

战术后方　tactical rear

战术决策　tactical decision

战役后方　operational rear

战役后方医院　campaign
　rear hospital

招聘　recruit

折旧　depreciation

折扣　discount

真实性;效度　validity

诊察费　diagnostic fee

诊断　diagnosis

诊断参照标准　reference standard
　of diagnosis

诊断符合率　consistency rate
　of diagnosis

诊断偏倚　diagnosis bias

诊断设备　diagnostic equipment

诊断相关组　diagnosis related groups
　（drg）

诊断治疗周期　diagnostic-
　therapeutic cycle

诊疗人次　number of visits

诊疗信息　the information of
　diagnosis and treatment

诊室　consulting room

阵亡　killed in action

争议　dispute

整合　integration

整群抽样　cluster sampling

整体服务系统　integrated delivery
　system（IDS）

整体护理　integrated nursing

整体护理质量评价　holistic care
　quality evaluation

整体计划　corporate plan

整体效应　holistic effect

整形外科　department of
　plastic surgery

整形外科医师　plastic surgeon

正常利润　normal profit

正常品　normal goods

正当程序　due process

正反馈　positive feedback

正规教育　regular education

正交设计　orthogonal design

正偏态分布　positive
　　skewness distribution

正式计划　formal planning

正式组织　formal organization

正态　normal

正态分布　normal distribution

正态性检验　normality test

证实性因子分析　confirmatory
　　factor analysis

证书　certification

政策法规　policy and code

政策分析　policy analysis

政策评价　policy evaluation

政策研究　policy research

政策影响分析　policy
　　impact analysis

政策主张　policy claim

政府补助　government subsidy

政府督导模式　government
　　supervision mode

政府法规　government regulation

政府公共关系　government
　　public relations

政府机构改革　reform of
　　government institutions

政府议案　government bill

政绩　administrative achievements

政委　commissar

政治部(处)主任　director of
　　political department

症状　symptom

支持系统　support system

支持型领导　supportive leadership

支出　payout

支付方式　payment system

支气管镜室　bronchoscope room

知名度　popularity；reputation

知情权　the right of awareness

知情人　informant

知情同意　informed consent

知识产权　intellectual property right
　　（IPR）

知识传递　knowledge transmission

知识更新　knowledge renewal

知识共享　information share

知识管理　knowledge management

知识获取　knowledge acquisition

知识结构   knowledge structure

知识经济   knowledge economy

知识流程   knowledge flow sheet

知识密集   knowledge denseness

执行层   execution level

执业药师   licensed pharmacist

执业药师   licensed pharmacists

执业医师   practicing doctor；
　　practicing physician

执业医师法   practicing
　　physicians law

直方图   histogram

直接成本   direct cost

直接经济负担   direct burden

直接人工   direct labor

直接融资   direct financing

直接投资   direct investment

直接效益   direct benefit

直线的;线性的   linear

直线回归   linear regression

直线趋势预测   linear forecasting

直线相关   linear correlation

职工   staff

职工福利   employee benefits

职工教育   employee education

职能科室   functional department

职位评价   position analysis

职务   duty

职务评审   duty evaluation

职业病   occupational disease

职业病预防   prevention of
　　occupational diseases

职业道德   professional ethics

职业康复   vocational rehabilitation

职业心理   occupational psychology

职业性白内障   occupational cataract

职业性哮喘   occupational asthma

指导型领导   instrumental leader

指定性后送   appointed evacuation

指挥   command

指数   exponential

指数平滑法   exponential
　　smoothing method

指数索赔量   exponential
　　claim amounts

指数原理   exponential principle

制裁   punish；sanction

制度   institution；system

制度安排   institutional arrangement

制度创新   system innovation

制度经济学   institutional economics

制度设计   institutional design

制度性保障   institutional guarantee

制衡机制   check-and-balance system

制约 restrict

治理机制 governing mechanism

治疗费 therapeutic fee

治疗设备 therapeutic equipment

治疗室 therapeutic room

治疗学 therapeutics

治愈 cure

治愈率 cure rate

质控室 quality control office

质量 quality

质量保证 quality assurance

质量保证体系 quality assurance system

质量标准 quality standard

质量策划 quality planning

质量调整生命年 quality adjusted life year（QALY）

质量方针 quality policy

质量改进 quality improvement

质量纲领 quality programs

质量管理 quality management

质量管理体系 quality management system

质量计划 quality plan

质量记录 quality records

质量监测；质量监督；质量监控 quality monitoring

质量检控 inspection and control of quality

质量检验 quality inspection

质量检验室 quality monitoring laboratory

质量控制 quality control

质量控制方法 quality control method

质量控制体系 quality control system

质量目标 quality objective

质量评定规则 rules for quality evaluation

质量评价 quality evaluation

质量认证 conformity certification

质量审核 quality audit

质量手册 quality manual

质量特性 quality characteristic

质量体系 quality system

质量体系认证 quality system certification

质量信息控制 quality information control

质量要求 quality requirements

质量一致性检验 inspection of quality conformity

质量诊断 quality diagnosis

质量证书　certificate of quality

质量指标　quality index

质量指标构建　establishment of quality index

质量仲裁　quality arbitration

质优价廉　good in quality and low in price

秩次　rank order

秩相关　rank correlation

智力　intelligence

智力资产　intelligent assets

智能　intelligence

智能化　intelligentization

智能决策支持系统　intelligent decision support system（IDSS）

滞纳金　fine for delaying payment

中等规模　medium scale

中国保监会　China Insurance Regulatory Commission

中国非处方药物协会　China Nonprescription Association（CNMA）

中国药典　Chinese Pharmacopoeia

中国药学会　Chinese Pharmaceutical Association

中国医疗器械质量认证中心　China quality certification center for medical devices

中国医药包装协会　China Pharmaceutical Packaging Association

中国制药装备行业协会　China Association for Pharmaceutical Equipment（CAPE）

中国中医研究院　China Academy of Traditional Chinese Medicine

中华人民共和国宪法　Constitution of the People's Republic of China

中华中医药学会　China Association of Chinese Medicine

中间产品　intermediate goods

中期规划　mid-term planning

中期预测　mid-term forecasting

中位生存时间　median survival time

中位数　median

中西医结合　combined Chinese and western medicine

中心功能检查室　central functional check room

中心手术室　central operating room

中心消毒供应室　central disinfection supply room

中心医院　central hospital

中药房　Chinese medicine pharmacy

中药师　Chinese medicine pharmacist

中药制剂室　Chinese medicine preparation laboratory

中医科　department of traditional Chinese medicine

中医师　doctor of traditional Chinese medicine

中医药　Chinese medicine

中医专业　specialty of Chinese medicine

中转医院　relay hospital

终末期肾病　end-stage renal disease（ESRD）

终末质量　terminal quality

终身保险　whole life insurance

终身学习　lifelong learning

终身追求　lifetime pursuit

肿瘤科　department of oncology

肿瘤科医师　oncologist

肿瘤医院　tumor hospital

仲裁　arbitration

重点学科　key discipline

重复测量研究　repeated measure study

重复测量资料　repeated measurement data

重复调查　repeated survey

重复横断面调查　repeated cross-sectional surveys

重复随访研究　repeated follow-up study

重复性　reproducibility

重伤室　severely wounded ward

重新评价　reevaluation

重症监护室　intensive care unit

周期时间　cycle length

主成分分析　principal components analysis

主动管理　active management

主动权　driving right

主动随访　active follow-up

主动性　activeness

主观预期效用　Subjective Expected Utility

主管部门　superintend department

主管护师　nurse-in-charge

主管技师　technologist-in-charge

主管药师　pharmacist-in-charge

主管中药师　Chinese drugs pharmacist in charge

主任办公室　director's office

主任护师　chief nurse-master

主任技师　chief technologist

主任科员　chief section member

主任药师　chief pharmacist

主任医师　chief physician

主效应　main effect

主治医师　doctor-in-charge

住房补贴　housing subsidies

住房分配　housing distribution

住房改革　housing reform

住房公积金制度　public housing funding system

住房津贴　housing allowance

住院　hospitalization

住院部　in-patient department

住院处　admitting office

住院服务　impatient services

住院患者　inpatient

住院人数　number of inpatients

住院申报　inpatient declaration

住院医师　resident physician

住宅　residential building

助教　teaching assistant

助理工程师　assistant engineer

助理员　assistant personnel

注射室　injection room

注资改制　capital injection and system reform

专家　specialist

专家评分法　specialist-scored method

专家预测　expert forecasting

专家咨询　expert consultation

专科护理　specialist care

专科医院　specialist hospital

专科治疗　specialized treatment

专利　patent

专门小组　panel

专题小组讨论　focus group discussion

专业化　specialization

专制式领导　autocratic leader

转变　transformation

转变政府职能　transform the government functions

转归　outcome

转换概率　transition probability

转诊中心　referral center

转制　transformation of operational system

准备金　reserve fund

准则效度　criterion-related validity

资本　capital

资本产出比率　capital output ratio

资本存量　capital stock

资本货物　capital goods

资本交易　capital transaction

资本平均产量　average product
　　of capital

资本消耗　capital consumption

资本影子价格　shadow price
　　of capital

资本运营规模　scale of
　　capital operation

资本运营战略　capital
　　operation strategy

资本支出　capital outlay

资本周转　capital turnover

资本主体　capital principal part

资产　assets

资产负债表　balance sheet

资产管理　asset management

资金短缺　capital shortage

资金管理　fund management

资料复印　data photocopy

资料收集　data collection

资料原件　original copy

资源　resource

资源管理　resource management

资源配置　resource allocation

资源误置　misallocation of resources

资源稀缺　resource scarcity

资源效率　resource efficiency

自变量　independent variable

自筹资金　funds raised by oneself

自动化　automatization

自动数据处理　automatic
　　data processing

自发　self-initiative

自发投资　spontaneous investment

自费　self-payment fee

自负盈亏　assume responsibility for
　　own profit and loss

自给自足　self-sufficiency

自救　self aid

自控　self-control

自然规律　natural law

自然垄断　natural monopoly

自然损耗　natural losses

自然系统　natural system

自然增长率　natural growth rate

自然资源　natural resource

自我保护意识　self-
　　protect consciousness

自我保健　self health care

自我超越　personal mastery

自我发展　self development

自我防御　ego-defense

自我积累　self-accumulation

自我控制法　self control

自我批评　self-criticism

自我实现　self-actualization

自我实现的需要　needs for
self-actualization

自我约束　self-restraint

自相关系数
autocorrelation coefficient

自信　confidence

自由度　degree of freedom（DF）

自由放任　laissez faire

自由进入　free entry

自由签约权　right of
free contracting

自由选择　freedom of choice

自愿　voluntary

自主管理　autonomous management

自主权　the right of autonomy

自主运营　independent operation

自组织　self-organization

自尊的需要　self-esteem need

综合管理体系　comprehensive
management system

综合竞争力　overall competitiveness

综合评比　comprehensive evaluation

综合评价法　comprehensive
evaluating method

综合数据处理系统　industrial

data processing

综合素质　comprehensive quality

综合性　comprehensiveness

综合医院　comprehensive hospital

综合预测
comprehensive forecasting

综合指标　comprehensive index

总保费　gross premium

总产量　total product

总成本　total cost

总额预算　global budget

总供给　aggregate supply

总固定成本　total fixed cost

总和生育率　total fertility rate

总后勤部卫生部　Medical
Department of General Logistics
Department of CPLA

总护士长　chief head nurse

总可变成本　total variable cost

总收益　total revenue

总体　population

总体健康感受　general
health perceptions

总体均衡　general equilibrium

总体医疗质量评价　general medical
quality evaluation

总务科　logistic office

总销售量　overall sales

总效用　total utility

总需求　aggregate demand

总医院　general hospital

总预算　overall budget

总则　general principle

总支出　total expenditure

纵向传播　vertical transmission

纵向调查　longitudinal survey

纵向公平　vertical equity

纵向联系　vertical relation

租金收入　rent revenue/income

租金支出　rent expense，rent

租赁　rent

组合化　combination

组合权重　combined weight

组内相关系数　intraclass correlation
coefficient（ICC）

组织　organization

组织变革　organizational reform

组织持续改进　continuous
improvement of the organization

组织管理　management
of organization

组织规模　size of the organization

组织间关系　inter-
organizational relations

组织结构　organizational structure

组织经济学
organizational economics

组织任务　organization mission

组织文化　organizational culture

组织行为学　organizational behavior

组织形象　organization image

组织愿景　organization vision

组织战略　organizational strategy

组织职能　organizational function

最大似然法　maximum likelihood

最大损失原理　maximal
loss principle

最大损失总额　maximal
aggregate loss

最低成本分析　minimum
cost analysis

最低工资　minimum wage

最低工资制度　minimum
wage system

最低生活保障
subsistence allowances

最低生活保障制度　system of
subsistence allowances

最高限额　ceiling

最高限价　price ceiling

最高责任限额　maximum

liability limit

最佳规模　optimal scale

最佳经济批量　best economic batch

最佳选择　optimal choice

最佳证据　best evidence

最佳资源配置　optimal

　　resource allocation

最小成本分析　cost

　　minimization analysis

最小二乘法　least sum of squares

最小库存余量　minimum balance

最优方案　optimal programme

最优价格　best price

最优可行　optimal feasible

最优控制　optimal control

最终产品　final goods

尊敬的需要　esteem needs

作业治疗师(士)

　　occupational therapist

作战区　combat zone

参 考 文 献

[1] 陆增琪.军事医学辞典[M].上海:上海辞书出版社,1997.

[2] 于春迟,刘爱春.柯林斯 COBUILD 英汉双解学习词典(精编版)[M].北京:外语教学与研究出版社,2007.

[3] 任真年.英汉现代医院质量管理词汇[M].北京:人民军医出版社,2003.

[4] 王发强,雷志勇.英汉、汉英医院管理学词汇[M].北京:人民军医出版社,1999.

[5] 郭志文.卫生勤务学词典[M].北京:人民军医出版社,1991.